THE DOCTOR'S BILL

THE
DOCTOR'S BILL

BY

HUGH CABOT

WITH AN INTRODUCTION BY
A. LAWRENCE LOWELL

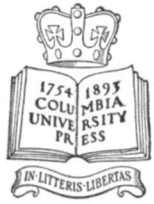

NEW YORK: MORNINGSIDE HEIGHTS

COLUMBIA UNIVERSITY PRESS

M · CM · XXXV

COPYRIGHT 1935
COLUMBIA UNIVERSITY PRESS

———

PUBLISHED 1935

PRINTED IN THE UNITED STATES OF AMERICA
BY QUINN & BODEN COMPANY, INC., RAHWAY, N. J.

To

THE CONSIDERABLE GROUP OF STUDENTS
OF MEDICINE WHO HAVE HONORED
ME BY THEIR CONFIDENCE

PREFACE

After more than thirty years of pretty intimate contact with medical students in various grades I am acutely aware that the undergraduate of today will have to take up his life's work in a very different environment from that in which I began. Since the beginning of the century not only have the economic and social conditions of the country changed, but science has so altered the practice of medicine that the physician entering practice today will offer a very different service and in a very different environment. My rather peripatetic habits have given me a perhaps better-than-average opportunity of seeing not only different types of students, but different types of practice, and in many parts of the country.

I find undergraduates and recent graduates very much alive to the new conditions, very eager for information, and very receptive to what one would like to call advice. I further observe that many of the physicians under forty are much puzzled, and although anxious to accommodate themselves to conditions as they are, find the adjustment difficult in view of the teaching and the opinion of their elders.

I am glad to be able to say that my former students still honor me by asking my advice, and I have been anxious to have something to offer them. I am very conscious, however, that they are the people who must "face the music" and not I. It is clear that most of the decisions which will ultimately affect their practice must be made by the younger group; but it is just possible that the generation to which I belong may help them by dint of having lived through the rapid changes which have led to the present confusion. We cannot do; but perhaps we may still be able to think. We should offer them our counsel, our judgment, and the results of our experience, but we must avoid handicapping them by our caution—which too often is but evidence of senile arteriosclerosis.

But the medical students and the younger physicians are not alone in asking, "Where do we go from here?" This is by no means a private battle, and anyone may get into it. The problems involved obviously invite study by the economist, statistician, the social scientist, as well as by the physician. Reverberations of their discussions have reached to the thinking public and will shortly reach to the Halls of Congress. There has been an immense amount of study undertaken by the above-mentioned groups. But, inevitably, each group—since it is made up of specialists—has had a different slant on the matter and has often overlooked what was common knowledge to one of the other groups.

The economist is likely to err upon the side of simplification. He tends to try to reduce the problem to the dimension of our old friend, the economic man. He tends to be a cold, detached person, apt to overlook the fact that the people affected by his plans are liable to be human beings, some of them even patients who may not be quite up to the niceties of balanced logic and theoretical economics. He has at times overlooked the possibly serious damage which might result to the atmosphere essential to the sound practice of medicine by the introduction of economic reforms which seem to him not only simple, but obvious.

The expert in social science has been likely to approach the whole problem from the side of poverty. He has been impressed by the results of poverty, by the crushing burden of living at all, under such economic conditions, in what may well seem to him a mad world. In fact most of the legislation which has been enacted—chiefly in other countries—in the attempt to obtain a more even distribution of satisfactory medical care, has approached the problem through the gateway of the relief of poverty. I do not suggest at all that this approach is not a desirable one. In fact, could the problems of poverty be solved, many of the difficulties of more equitable distribution of medical care would by that act disappear. On the other hand, the setting up of a plan for medical care as part of a program for the relief of poverty has, at least in other countries, resulted in legislation which has required frequent and often drastic amendment to make it work at all.

The physician obviously approaches the problem in a preferred position. He, at least, is grounded in a knowledge of disease and its management. Physicians are certainly the qualified experts to whom the community must look for guidance on questions of a technical nature. But even physicians have had considerable difficulty in seeing the whole field. They are, and must be, from the very nature of their calling intense individualists. To them Medicine still retains—thank God—some of the qualities of a religion. They take fright at the thought that profane hands may soil the Temple of their God—Service. At this point emotion is likely to come into action and understanding goes out of the door. Furthermore, they have a very real vested interest which it would not be human in them to disregard. Often enough in their opposition to change they have failed to grasp the implications of the profound economic and social changes which have been going on about them. As a result, on too many occasions they have fought a series of futile rear-guard actions which have left them still on the defensive.

Finally, there is the controlling interest of the public, who, for better or worse, cannot avoid being profoundly affected by any action which may result from the cogitations of the three groups previously mentioned. Here again point of view enters on the scene. Since we live today in a thoroughly commercialized world, it is often difficult for the average man to grasp the process of mind which lies behind the bill which he receives for medical services. He cannot see why he should have to pay more than did his friend, Jones, for what appears to him to be the same article. He cannot grasp the intricacies of the sliding scale in medical fees—and indeed he is in good company.

The task which I have set myself is to give some account of the background from which the problem of adjusting modern medical practice to the requirements of the community has emerged, to present its economic setting, to set forth the various methods which have been employed in other countries in attacking similar situations, and, if possible, to suggest the principles upon which we must rely in working out for ourselves a proper course to steer in what is, in many respects, an uncharted sea. Now it may well be that I am disqualified at the outset because I belong to an obviously interested group. In fact a good friend of mine—though a Doctor of Philosophy—has already expressed to me his opinion that no Doctor of Medicine can present the case fairly. To this I am inclined to enter the plea of *nolo contendere*.

In attempting to make reasonably understandable the various economic and financial aspects of the problem I have inevitably had recourse to factual studies, few of which are entirely contemporary. It will perhaps be suggested that different and more recent figures would warrant a very different conclusion. This I am not at all inclined to deny, but I insist that the sort of basic assumptions upon which plans for the future must be based can never rest firmly upon statistical fact. Unfortunately facts "keep no better than fish." No matter what array of statistical evidence we put forward, it will certainly be untrue in whole or in part very shortly. It is not statistical fact but tendency with which we must be concerned. We are not attempting to plan for the moment, but for the future. If we can make clear to ourselves what tendencies are indicated as probable as a result of the prolongation of lines of change which we can see foreshadowed in the more recent past, we are more likely to obtain a sound foundation than if we place too great reliance upon contemporary fact. Mere factual knowledge will not save us, for there are few conclusions so unlikely that they cannot be supported by statistical evidence. What we need is not knowledge, but wisdom, that essence extracted from fact as a result of sound thinking.

That a satisfactory working solution of the present confused situation is of the first importance will not require demonstration. It is perhaps true that the continuance of any given civilization is more importantly influenced by its ability to protect itself against the diseases and accidents to which it gives rise than by any other single factor. If we should allow the development of medical science to outstrip by any great distance our ability to supply medical care in practical measure to the great majority of the population, then we have at least weakened one of the important supports upon which civilization rests.

Equally obviously, as I think, the solution will require good-tempered, patient, and receptive discussion by several groups of experts. In their own field the physicians can supply the evidence, but they cannot be expected to supply the mature judgment in the economic, social, and financial fields, which will obviously be important and probably essential to success. Too often in the discussions which have taken place, particularly in this country and during the last ten years, these requirements have been lacking. Too often one group has become impatient with the other. Still more frequently one group has assumed its ability to deal with expert questions quite out of its own field. Since we are concerned with the offering of sound service to the whole population, it is essential that we should bring to the task the best thinkers in the various fields and that no conclusions, upon which we propose to act, should be arrived at by *ex parte* discussion.

I have decided to use, as a title for this book, *The Doctor's Bill*. This seems, on the whole, to suggest, as well as may be, what I am trying to say. It will be noted in this and kindred discussions that the problem of the "bill" is constantly recurring. We could do *so* much better if we could solve this problem of the bill, which so regularly turns up either from the doctor or on his behalf. The title may also be construed in a quasi-legal sense as indicating a bill-of-particulars in the case now coming before the bar of Public Opinion in the guise of The People vs. The Care of Their Health.

I desire here to acknowledge the stimulating assistance of Professor Ernest L. Bogart and the many helpful suggestions of Professor Douglass V. Brown, upon both of whom I inflicted the manuscript. To Dean Willard C. Rappleye I am under great obligation for help on this and many other occasions. Particularly I wish to express my profound gratitude to my secretary, Geraldine Timpayne, for her untiring energy, patience, accuracy, and complete understanding.

Hugh Cabot

ROCHESTER, MINNESOTA
MARCH 29, 1935

CONTENTS

PREFACE	vii
INTRODUCTION BY A. LAWRENCE LOWELL	xv
I. MEDICAL PRACTICE IN 1890 AND IN 1930	3
II. MODERN MEDICAL DIAGNOSIS AND ITS REQUIREMENTS	21
III. OUR MEDICAL RESOURCES	35
IV. THE GENERAL PRACTICE OF MEDICINE	50
V. SPECIALISTS AND GROUP MEDICINE	64
VI. GROUP HEALTH SERVICES	79
VII. THE WORKMEN'S COMPENSATION ACTS	94
VIII. THE INCOME OF PHYSICIANS	114
IX. THE ABILITY TO PAY FOR ILLNESS	132
X. HEALTH INSURANCE IN CONTINENTAL EUROPE	141
XI. HEALTH INSURANCE IN THE BRITISH ISLES	158
XII. MEDICAL NEEDS IN THE UNITED STATES	180
XIII. SOME SUGGESTED METHODS OF IMPROVEMENT	207
XIV. LAISSEZ FAIRE OR COMPULSION	224
XV. WHERE DO WE GO FROM HERE?	252
NOTES	285
BIBLIOGRAPHY	293
INDEX	301

INTRODUCTION

Hugh Cabot has asked me to write an introduction to this book, and although as incompetent as any non-medical man must be to discuss the questions raised therein, I am very glad to do so because I have long known him and greatly admired his character and career, his courage, and his clearness in seeing the essential points in any matter to which he turns his attention.

Graduating from the Harvard Medical School in 1898, he built up a practice in his special field of genito-urinary surgery, but abandoned it in 1916 to take charge of a British surgical base hospital, which he commanded throughout the war, doing an amazing amount of work for the initial equipment of his plant. Returning three years later with his private practice in Boston evaporated, he was appointed Professor of Surgery and later Dean of the Medical School at the University of Michigan, and Chief Surgeon of the new hospital being built there. Fearless as ever, he lost this position after ten years chiefly because he strove, against the opposition of many in the profession there, to carry out in the hospital principles which he considered essential in a tax-supported institution of such a nature. Since that time he has been a member of the Mayo Clinic at Rochester, Minnesota.

Now in regard to this book, which is the product of long and discriminating observation. The advance of knowledge has thrown upon the scrap heap many processes useful in their day, but nowhere else has this been so true as in medicine and surgery. Chemical, bacterial and microscopic analysis has revolutionized diagnosis; knowledge of the secretions of the ductless and other glands, and of the functions of the blood and tissues, has brought new elements into the treatment of disease; anesthetics and antiseptics have made surgery a different art.

In his first chapter, on medical practice in 1890 and 1930, Dr. Cabot points out in a striking way the effect of such changes on the position of the physician. The period is substantially that of his own experience from medical school onward, and with characteristic fairness he portrays the loss as well as the gain in the superseding of the former family physician, ignorant of methods since learned, but familiar with personal and hereditary peculiarities of his patients.

In the following chapters he discusses the application of modern medicine to present needs, its effect on diagnosis, on the number, training and distribution of physicians, the enormous growth and auxiliary use of hospitals, the diversity in lines of practice with the income of the several types of physicians, the total cost to the community and the ability of the public to pay. The plan is logical, and proceeds with a survey of the various methods of health insurance in Europe and their applicability here, a study of our own needs, of how some industrial concerns have tried to meet them, and, finally, of the sundry methods suggested for improving medical service throughout this country.

His estimates of the systems adopted in European nations, with their merits and defects, is sympathetic and impartial; and he is not misled, as many people are, by the utility of something in a foreign land, into thinking that because it may work well there it can be transplanted bodily to another soil with similar results. Our conditions, he feels, and hence our problems, are, *sui generis*, to be examined as such; and he discusses them with an open mind, not hesitating to criticize the medical profession for its shortcomings, its lapses into a commercial attitude and its lack of interest in the larger aspects of its potential functions. From his experience he perceives the benefits of the Mayo Clinic, to which he now belongs; and he evidently thinks that in organizations of that type lies much hope for the future. Of course, he desires universal medical service of the best grade, and recognizes that if the public wants such a service it must be ready to pay what it costs, while the profession must be redeemed from the temptation to commercialism, and must be able to earn an income reasonable in view of the length and expense of the training.

The book should be read, not only by the physicians, but also by laymen who want to know the questions confronting the treatment of individual and public health. No one need fear technical terms or obscurity; for it is not a treatise on disease, but a discussion on broad lines of its social aspects.

A. Lawrence Lowell

THE DOCTOR'S BILL

I

MEDICAL PRACTICE IN 1890 AND IN 1930

A clear picture of the present relation of the practice of medicine to society will be best obtained if we can put it in its proper historical setting. The practice of medicine is no more static than any other field of endeavor, and a clear picture cannot be obtained by looking at it at any particular point in its development. It is not enough to appreciate that medical practice has changed. We must also get some notion of the rate of change as compared with that in other activities. But, before we can do this, we must note the varying rate of change in world conditions as a whole, and appreciate that progress and change have proceeded at very different rates at different periods. The situation was concisely stated by Whitehead.[1] He clearly showed that up to 1870 changes in economic and social conditions had taken place so slowly that it was a fair assumption that a man's grandchildren would live under conditions substantially similar to those under which he, himself, had lived. Since that time change has taken place so rapidly as to bring such an assumption into violent contradiction with the facts. From this, of course, flow two consequences: first, that adjustments between professional activities, such as the practice of medicine, and current social and economic conditions will have to be made much more frequently and perhaps more profoundly; and second, that any attempt to predict the future will have to be confined to a period of time much shorter than was safe at a previous period. On the other hand, it is important to appreciate that all progress in such fields is predicated upon the assumption of some accuracy of prediction over a reasonable period, and that while the periods for which prediction is safe and upon which action can be based have been severely contracted, we must nevertheless continue to make predictions and to act upon them.

THE PRACTICE OF MEDICINE ABOUT 1890

In attempting to draw a picture of medical practice about 1890 it is important to indicate what was then the condition of medical education and what was the extent of knowledge with which the practitioner was equipped. At that time medical education in this country was finally concluding its emergence from the apprentice system which had held sway since Colonial days. In the earlier period medical education had consisted in the taking of certain courses of lectures, which included some knowledge of the elementary principles of physics, chemistry, and biology, followed by the dogmatic, didactic presentation of the accepted doctrines of diagnosis and treatment. This was followed by an apprenticeship, either to an active practitioner or in the form of "walking the hospital," in which students attached themselves to eminent physicians having hospital opportunities and learned from them by precept and example the current medical doctrines. During the thirty years precedent to 1890 the definitely educational courses in medicine had been steadily expanded and at that time covered a period of three years. The practice of attending the same lectures for more than one year had disappeared, and a graded course had come into being, coupled with increasing use of clinical lectures and the more simple laboratory experiments. The course, however, was relatively brief as compared with the present time, and few of the students had any previous college training. Nevertheless, the course was adequate to familiarize the students with the more important settled facts in the underlying sciences, and to give them reasonable clinical experience. At the end of this course—which, curiously enough, led to a doctor's degree quite out of line with academic practice in other fields—the student commonly entered directly into general practice and slowly built up a clientele as his experience justified people in relying upon him. A moderate number of students in comfortable circumstances were able to include a course of study in Europe—generally in Germany, Austria, or France. The amount of knowledge of the sciences underlying medicine, and the amount of special knowledge in the various fields of medicine, was not up to that time so great but that it could be grasped, at least to some extent, by a single mind. Practically all the physicians were general practitioners, the only specialists being in the fields of the eye, ear, nose, and throat—and even they commonly combined their special practice with general practice. Indeed, the distinguished surgeons of that day frequently continued to see patients in the general medical field, and specialization such as is common today was almost unknown.

Although in those days, as at the present time, effective treatment necessarily had to be based upon accurate diagnosis, the methods by which anything approaching scientific accuracy could be obtained were rather meager. Diagnosis was still largely based upon physical examination supplemented by a few instruments of precision, such as the thermometer and, to some extent, the microscope. The stethoscope was in common use, yet one would frequently see a most distinguished physician of the day discard this instrument and apply his ear directly to the patient's chest wall, though with a towel interposed. This meant, of course, that they were still relatively distrustful of the newfangled stethoscope and preferred to trust to what they could hear with their ear applied to the chest. That the intervening towel, commonly used partly for delicacy and partly for protection, seriously interfered with their interpretation of sounds need be noted only in passing.

Applied chemistry and bacteriology were of a relatively simple character. Examination of the urine was commonly confined to its appearance, reaction, presence or absence of albumin, specific gravity, and a somewhat cursory microscopic examination of the sediment. Bacteriology was still a young science not widely applied and often regarded with distrust. In a word, the practitioners of that day depended upon the use of their five senses, which were often very highly developed by practice and experience. As an example may be cited the amount of information which they gleaned from an examination of the tongue, which did in fact give them information that the medical student of today would regard with distrust and that even the experienced practitioner of the present time would be incapable of obtaining. These men were quite as skillful as, and perhaps more skillful than, their modern successors in eliciting information by observation and palpation. With them prolonged experience was a great asset, and the tendency of the time to rely upon senior practitioners rather than upon the younger men was based upon the fact that by contact with a large number of patients they had gradually developed skill in noting and weighing the importance of various clinical signs and symptoms, which at times amounted almost to deified guesswork. Experience, boldness, and character were at a premium. Profound scientific knowledge, familiarity with science, and the ability to assign the proper weight to facts obtained by the application of the scientific method were not for them. Accurate diagnosis had commonly to wait upon time, and often enough the patient would be either well or dead before an opinion, probably accurate, could be expressed. This required the continuance of "the cloak of mystery" which so frequently characterized the practice of an earlier day. Certainty was uncommon, and frequently a course of treatment based upon suppositions was successful only because the patient survived it. To some extent there still persisted a certain religious atmosphere in relation to the practice of medicine. One frequently found distinguished practitioners arguing with each other not upon a basis of fact, but upon a basis of faith, and defending their faiths with true religious fervor. This was very strikingly shown in the opposition which arose to the teachings of Lord Lister in regard to the possibility of controlling infection in wounds.

One remembers that this was the day when appendicitis, which has now become a household pet, was still unknown and patients suffered from, and died of, inflammation of the bowels or even perityphlitis when in fact they had acute suppurative appendicitis. (One may assume that it was comforting to the family that the patient should die of some disease with a long name. This, however, did not interfere with the common practice of dying.) It was still the day when patients "went into a decline," which often was but a manifestation of rapidly spreading tuberculosis. Diphtheria was but little understood and still masqueraded as croup. It was of mysterious origin and its occurrence in a family was often attended with drenching of the drainage system with peppermint in order to discover leaks. That the repair of such leaks in plumbing was desirable cannot be denied, but that it had no important effect in freeing the atmosphere from the bacillus of diphtheria may be confidently asserted. Typhoid fever was a disease of enormous frequency, particularly in centers of population, and its connection with faulty drainage and contaminated water supply was yet to be clearly faced by the community. In some parts of the country yellow fever still took its toll and was regarded as of miasmic origin. Over a larger area malaria was still thought related to the damp of the evening, and not to the bite of the ubiquitous and commonly infected mosquito. Even I recall vividly the discussions which arose over the appearance of malaria along the Charles River—that beautiful, if boggy, stream meandering in the environs of Boston. Its advent came quite promptly after the extensive removal of gravel from the banks of the river, some distance from Boston, for the purpose of filling the unornamental bog of the so-called Back Bay. The occurrence of malaria was charged to the releasing of noxious miasms by overturning of the soil, and it was some years later before it became clearly understood that the appearance of malaria in that section could be traced directly to the importation of Italian laborers who quite unintentionally endowed the mosquitoes with the plasmodia of malaria which they, in turn, kindly passed on to the pleasure-seeking folk intent upon canoeing on the river after the sun was low. One should remember also the prevalence of what was called scrofula, being in fact a form of tuberculosis—the connection of which with the milk of tuberculous cows was, of course, unknown. Abdominal surgery, which today bulks so large in the more violent fields of therapeutics known as surgery, was then a relatively modest development. The Listerian doctrine of wound infection was not yet fully developed, and the opening of the abdomen was still a ceremony surrounded by much pomp and circumstance and attended with the slopping of antiseptic solutions into the wound. That these solutions were life-saving does not prevent our recognizing that they did considerable damage to the tissues in the process of eliminating or curtailing infection. The surgery of other fields was still, relatively speaking, in its infancy. Operations upon bones and upon joints were still regarded as hazardous undertakings. The invasion of the more remote cavities of the body, such as those lying within the skull, was undertaken only for the most urgent reasons. No accurate preoperative knowledge could be obtained in regard to conditions lying within the abdomen, and knowledge of diseases of the urinary tract was almost wholly guesswork.

The development of hospitals as an aid in the practice of medicine was still in its infancy. Probably most of the hospitals in the country at that time either belonged to the almshouse group or were for the care of the insane. The great charity hospitals had, of course, been developed and were playing an important part, but they were relatively few in number and patterned after the great voluntary hospitals of Great Britain. The time was not sufficiently removed from the day of the so-called hospital diseases—hospital gangrene, erysipelas, septicemia, and child bed fever—to inspire people with great confidence in hospital care. It was well within the memory of most people when to enter a hospital with any surgical wound was more likely to be followed by death than recovery. It was more or less well known that the probability of recovery under such circumstances was better at home than in a hospital. People still regarded hospitals as places where a great many went in and very many less came out. Only for those who could not afford to die at home were hospitals regarded as proper places in which to die. This must not of course be taken as evidence that the great charity hospitals situated, chiefly, in the larger cities were of little account as great storehouses of wisdom and important laboratories for the application and development of modern knowledge. It should be superfluous to point out that from hospital practice has developed much of our present ability to apply science to the diagnosis and treatment of disease, however, in those days demonstration of this had just begun, and for people in comfortable or moderate circumstances the hospital was often a last resort. Even in my earlier days, just before the beginning of the present century, the majority of surgical operations were undertaken in private houses. That this resulted in standing the whole domestic arrangement upon its head was perhaps an advantage in that it lent an air of importance and dignity to the proceeding. In those days one still persisted in tearing up carpets, taking down pictures, and washing floors, mop boards and walls with corrosive sublimate—considerably to their disadvantage and probably only occasionally endangering the bacteria, which were erroneously supposed to be subdued by this process. That the whole proceeding had its largest effect in stirring up whatever dust might be present was commonly overlooked. There was a lack of clear appreciation of the fact that most infection in surgical operations comes from the surgeon, his associates, or his paraphernalia—including his tools of trade, his sponges, and his dressings. However, it was notoriously true that the incidence of wound infection clearly attributable to the operation itself was importantly lower in this kind of house-to-house surgery than in the wards of the great charity hospitals.

Social and Economic Conditions

Important changes have taken place in social and economic conditions during the last forty years. In 1890 the distribution of population was importantly different, though the tendency of people to collect in large cities was, of course, well established and proceeding rapidly. Industry had grown to occupy a very important position, and yet it was still true that nearly two-thirds of the population was rural, living in relatively small and sometimes isolated communities. In 1890 the urban population was 22,298,359, while the rural population was 40,649,355. Outside of the large centers of population the independent workman, the small storekeeper, and the artisan were still relatively numerous, constituting, with the farmer, a relatively large number of people who could not be properly classified as wage-earners, and who were relatively independent. It is to be noted also that the farmer had not at that period graduated into the capitalist class. He was still to a considerable extent a person who lived on the land, primarily as a method of supporting his family, and who sold his surplus crop at the neighboring four-corner village. The days were yet to come of enormous farms, capitalized, sometimes grossly beyond their value, operated importantly or largely by machinery and employing relatively few people to do the work. A beginning had been made in the transportation of labor to the western country to "get in the crop," and at the time there was the beginning of what later developed into a very important seasonal migration for that purpose. In industry the great combinations later called trusts were still in their infancy. Many of the industrial hazards and diseases resulting from elaborate industrial processes were either nonexistent or unrecognized. Transportation was a very different matter from what it is today. The great transcontinental railroads had been built. In the eastern part of the country, where industrial development had gone further, railroad transportation was relatively satisfactory, but for much of the country no such methods were available. Roads, except the main highways, were, as a rule, unsatisfactory, and the latter were not good judged by any standard of the last quarter of a century. The automobile was, of course, unknown. The doctor used the horse as his motive power, utilizing the buggy or chaise, but in a not inconsiderable area he had to travel on horseback with saddlebags. The telephone was in its infancy; its development—which may be judged to be both a boon and a nuisance—was yet to come. From all this it is evident that the physician's radius of action was relatively small, that the time consumed in making visits even in his neighborhood was excessive, as judged by modern standards, and that should a journey of more than twenty-five or thirty miles be necessary, a whole day might well be spent on the undertaking. Under these circumstances it was commonly difficult to apply even the then existing scientific aids to diagnosis, and in the vast majority of cases the diagnosis had to be made, and the treatment carried out, on the basis of a physical examination utilizing the doctor's senses, the clinical thermometer, and the stethoscope. The amount of time consumed in transportation made it difficult or impossible for the physician to see his patients with a frequency which might have been desirable, nor could he keep in touch with them by telephone. In this connection it should be recalled that the supply of trained nurses was still meager, and the great assistance given by them in the oversight and reporting of changes and symptoms was not usually available.

On the other hand, certain advantages which were associated with this type of distribution of population, and with the relatively inadequate transportation, have today been severely curtailed. This was the heyday of the family physician, who, situated in a town or village, generally knew every member of the families which he attended, might have at least a bowing acquaintance with most of the population, and thus be in possession of an amount and variety of information concerning family tendencies and habits, mental and physical, which were of inestimable value not only in diagnosis but, perhaps more importantly, in prognosis. As an illustration of what I mean, I may tell the story of a consultation at which I assisted as late as the beginning of the present century of which an aunt of mine was the subject. It was attended by two professors of medicine at Harvard, a professor of surgery at the same institution—who still enjoyed a reputation as a medical diagnostician—and the family physician. The lady was adjudged to have an extensive consolidation of the right lung, the typical lobar pneumonia of that period. She was apparently in the fourth or fifth day of the disease, the temperature and pulse were not abnormal, and her condition seemed satisfactory. The experts, having conducted their examinations, retired, as was the custom, to another room to discuss diagnosis, prognosis, and treatment. They agreed as to the diagnosis, regarded the prognosis as on the whole favorable, and had little to suggest in the way of treatment. At this point it occurred to one of them to ask the opinion of the family physician to find whether he concurred in their well-considered views. He remarked tersely that the lady was a Jones before she married; that Joneses who showed abdominal distension on the fourth or fifth day of a pneumonia died; and that she would die within the week. She did. This illustrates the immense value of knowledge of family characteristics, not only possible but common in that day, which has become increasingly difficult, or impossible, with the rapid shifting of population.

In the same connection I remember consulting a general practitioner of wide knowledge in a suburb of Boston in regard to a member of a family whom he had treated for years and whom I had seen on account of attacks of abdominal pain of no very distinctive character. I admitted that I was puzzled, and with the machinery then available for diagnosis was unable to convict any of his internal organs of criminal tendencies. He then said to me, "Oh, I have known the family for years. The Smiths always have belly-aches and they never amount to anything." His opinion proved correct.

The equipment of the physician of that day did not need to be elaborate, and could generally be carried in the "doctor's bag" of the period. He would need his stethoscope, his clinical thermometer, and a fair assortment of pills for more or less emergency use. If he were engaged in obstetrical practice he would require his obstetrical forceps, and he commonly had with him a small assortment of surgical instruments such as could be carried in a pocket case.

We may thus summarize the situation by pointing out that the practitioner of that day did not have at his command most of the scientific methods of accurate diagnosis which are today available, that he was far more dependent upon his five senses, and that his value as a physician depended more upon wide and prolonged experience than is the case today. His radius of activity was much more limited. The number of people whom he could actually see in a day was relatively small; the frequency with which he could visit them was much reduced; and, lacking the medium of the telephone, he could not get information in regard to patients whom he was unable to visit. To some extent counterbalancing this was the possibility of his having long and intimate knowledge of the individuals concerned. Not infrequently he might have assisted into the world all the children in a given family and continue for years to have them under his care. Of course, this was of inestimable value. It did, in fact, enable the family physician to be of considerable service in the then undeveloped fields of preventive medicine and social service, and, what was more important, it enabled him to put any particular illness in its proper setting as concerns heredity, social, and economic conditions. He was in a position to be, and was in many instances, the wise counsellor of the family on many questions not, accurately speaking, concerned with disease. When we recall that, at least in recent times, something like one-half of the conditions concerning which a physician is consulted will prove to be due, not to some ailment properly labeled as a disease, but to maladjustment, or lack of adjustment, in social, economic, and moral matters, we can readily see that the family physician of that era, in spite of his handicaps in obtaining accurate knowledge, might well be a most important factor in the management of the public health.

The Practice of Medicine about 1930

Though it is probably unnecessary, in order to keep the record clear, it may be wise to recall that the development of scientific knowledge during the forty years under survey has given us more new knowledge, some of which is applicable to the treatment of disease, than the whole previous period of recorded history put together. The accumulation of scientific fact literally staggers the imagination, and it is probably true that part of our confusion of the present day is due to our inability to digest, arrange, and correlate these facts with the business of everyday living. Forty years ago the physician could keep himself relatively abreast of increasing knowledge if he had at his disposal—as was frequently not the case—a very moderate supply of medical publications. Today it is probably within the facts to state that should the physician undertake to be really familiar with the new knowledge which may become applicable to the treatment of disease he would have to spend the greater part, if not the whole, of his time in reading current publications. Even were he in a position to do this, he would probably lack the time necessary to digest this knowledge, and certainly lack the opportunity for what used to be called contemplation—a process of mind not fashionable today. It will not be possible to review even hastily the amount of accumulated knowledge bearing upon the treatment of disease which has developed during the present century. At best, we can only refer to the fields and suggest some of the applications of this knowledge now required of the physician. While it has always been true that the practice of medicine was an attempt to apply knowledge in more or less scientific fields to the treatment of disease, it has remained for the present century to develop those fields to such an extent that modern science can not only be applied, but is absolutely essential to the obtaining of those facts which must ultimately underlie accurate diagnosis and, consequently, all sound plans for treatment. The extent to which the sciences, loosely referred to as the fundamental sciences underlying the practice of medicine, have been made available almost beggars description. Parenthetically, one may point out that though the physician is likely to think of these sciences as contributing to his art, they are of course independent sciences in which investigation is steadily going on and in which much of the knowledge obtained is not apparently applicable to the practice of medicine. One must briefly review the developments of bacteriology, physiology, pathology, pharmacology, physics, and chemistry, to say nothing of anatomy, in order to appreciate the extent to which the new knowledge in these fields has altered the outlook of the physician and, perhaps more important, the requirements placed upon him if he is to bring to his patient all of the assistance which is available.

BACTERIOLOGY

Bacteriology was a young science forty years ago, and relatively few of its discoveries were sufficiently complete to be available. True, the bacillus of tuberculosis had been isolated and was a matter of general knowledge. However, the application of that knowledge to the diagnosis and treatment of disease was still rudimentary. The organisms concerned with diphtheria, pneumonia, typhoid fever—to mention only a few—were unknown. The parasites causing malaria, hookworm, amoebic dysentery, were yet to be discovered. The spirillum causing syphilis was unknown. With the growth of knowledge in the field of bacteriology, and springing from it, came the development of serology and an understanding of the processes of immunity. Thus, in the field of diagnosis, the Widal reaction, a characteristic reaction of the blood during typhoid fever, and the Wassermann reaction, a reaction of the blood in the presence of syphilis, became of outstanding importance. In the field of treatment sera for the control of diphtheria, meningitis, and pneumonia have been developed, and, perhaps most important, in the field of preventive medicine vaccination or inoculation has been worked out to produce immunity against typhoid fever, diphtheria, and scarlet fever. At the earlier period vaccination against smallpox alone was known. This list is brief and intended only to be suggestive; it could be widely extended.

PATHOLOGY

Pathology was referred to in that day as morbid anatomy and, though far more developed than bacteriology, was still young. The mechanical methods of preparing very thin sections of tissue, the methods of staining these so as to bring out their peculiar appearances and characteristics were in an early stage of development. The possibility of removing a piece of tissue apart from or at the time of a surgical operation, and submitting it for immediate examination, a report of which could be made in five, or at most, ten, minutes was unknown. More recently, as the result of the removal of portions or the whole of a tumor, the possibility of grading tumors as to their degree of malignancy has affected not only the ability of the physician to predict the progress of malignant disease but to some extent so to alter the treatment as to increase the possibility of alleviation or cure. Without going into superfluous detail, it will be sufficiently obvious that the development of pathology has made accurate diagnosis more or less immediately available, and guesswork has to that extent been transformed into certainty. During this forty-year period has grown up the greater part of our knowledge of the peculiarities of the blood, a field now referred to as hematology. Examinations of the blood are now of outstanding, or even of absolutely essential, importance in the diagnosis of many conditions, and are frequently resorted to as guides in treatment. Thus, various diseases of the blood, such as pernicious anemia and various leukemias, previously diagnosed inaccurately or not at all, can now be discovered with great certainty. The diagnosis of malaria depends upon finding in the blood the parasite causing the disease. Accurate counts of various constituents of the blood are constantly required in diagnosis, and the increase of certain of the white blood cells is of importance in estimating the severity of, and the reactions to, various infections. In fact, hematology has become a developed and very important branch of laboratory science.

PHARMACOLOGY

In the field of our knowledge in regard to drugs enormous advances have been made. Pharmacology has become a science, and the tendency of the earlier day to administer drugs in enormous or infinitesimal doses with a rather vague knowledge of the probable action, together with the tendency to administer many pharmaceutical combinations which were probably without effect except upon the mind of the patient, has been severely curtailed. Pharmacology, using the machinery of chemistry, has run to earth the active principles of many of the drugs. Using the machinery of physiology, it has been able to test their action with the result that many noxious potions of an earlier day have been relegated to the limbo of the unknown. Accurate dosage using the active principles of drugs which in the past contained a large proportion of worthless or actually objectionable constituents has become possible. Again, using the machinery of chemistry it has been possible to produce synthetically, and consequently with accuracy, many drugs which previously had to be extracted laboriously, and in impure form, from vegetable compounds. To pharmacology should be credited the development of so-called intravenous therapy, by which accurate quantities of solutions may be introduced directly into the circulation. That this has resulted in some curtailment of the number of drugs administered is clearly an advantage, but its greatest achievement is that dosage has come within the limits of scientific accuracy and the physician may today count with certainty upon the effects of much of his treatment, which at the earlier day were highly problematical.

PHYSIOLOGY

It is almost literally true that the physician who learned his physiology prior to 1890 or even prior to the beginning of this century would find himself almost completely unaquainted with the modern views in that field. In few branches of science have more important and far-reaching advances been made. Though many of the older conceptions have not been wholly superseded, they have been elaborated and extended almost beyond recognition. Part of the advance, at least, has been due to the possibility of applying other forms of scientific development to the study, such as the use of X rays in studying the function of the intestine in animals. Knowledge of the function of the brain has been importantly extended. Most of the present knowledge in regard to the behavior and functions of the gastro-intestinal tract has come since that time. Using the newer methods supplied by physics and chemistry, knowledge of respiration and the part played by the various elements in the nervous system, more particularly the so-called autonomic portion, has been enormously advanced. Again using the assistance of chemistry, knowledge of the physiology of the kidney, liver, and pancreas has been highly developed, and one should also mention the increased knowledge of the various ductless glands—the adrenal, thyroid, parathyroid, ovary, and so forth. These advances have to a large extent rebuilt the foundations upon which much diagnosis and, consequently, much treatment was based.

PHYSICS

The contributions of physics to the development of modern medicine have been very great. Space will only permit a few of them to be suggested. Very far-reaching developments have followed the discovery and development of the X ray, both in diagnosis and in treatment. Allied to this was the discovery of radium and its uses. The application of the electric light with a so-called cold filament has made possible the construction of instruments permitting examination of the cavities of the body; among such apparatus should be mentioned the ophthalmoscope, the otoscope, the bronchoscope, and the cystoscope. To physics should also be credited the development of the electrocardiograph, an instrument of real importance in the diagnosis of obscure diseases of the heart. Physics has also contributed very importantly to the therapeutic field through increased knowledge of heat and light, making possible very fundamental and far-reaching developments in the field referred to as physiotherapy. In a word, many of the instruments of precision now essential to modern physical diagnosis have come about through developments of modern physics.

CHEMISTRY

Many of the most revolutionary changes in the management of disease are based upon the developments of modern chemistry. Our still very incomplete knowledge of the changes going on within the body, referred to under the general heading of metabolism, depends upon modern knowledge of biochemistry. Much advance has been made in our knowledge of the chemistry of digestion. All of the modern important tests of kidney function rest upon a chemical basis, as do the determinations of basal metabolic rates useful in the management of diseases of the thyroid gland and in various other situations. Our still vague knowledge of the function of the liver has developed to its present level on the basis of chemistry, and it may be confidently asserted that further, more complete knowledge will soon be forthcoming.

The list might be extended almost indefinitely, but it is only important to indicate to what extent the modern basis of medicine rests upon science, and the essential importance for the physician of understanding an immense amount of knowledge not available to his predecessor forty years ago. It might also be suggested at this time that a recognition by the public of the essential importance of such knowledge will make easier the comprehension of the increased, and probably increasing, requirements in medical education. This might lead to a more sympathetic understanding of the forces underlying specialization, since it should be at once evident that the human mind is incapable of grasping and keeping continuously familiar with all the developments of science likely to be applicable to medicine, and at the same time carry on an active medical practice.

Equipment of the Modern Physician

It should be clear that the modern physician will require a very different and much larger amount of equipment, both physical and intellectual, than that properly required forty years ago. At the earlier period it was commonly true that the physician shared with the minister and the lawyer the distinction of being the best educated man in his community. This was particularly true of the smaller communities, which contained in that day considerably more than half of the population. Today the physician enjoys no such distinction. With the tendency of people to gather together in large centers, he now finds himself surrounded by a large number of people who are quite his equals in education.

This is neither the time nor the place to discuss in detail the requirements of modern medical education, but it may be proper to suggest that he who is to pass judgment upon the applicability of various developments of science to the care and treatment of patients, who is to assay the weight to be given to an assortment of scientific fact which may be gathered together for the accurate diagnosis of any particular condition, and, especially, who is to assist his patients in their struggle to maintain their balance in a confusing, almost bewildering civilization, must needs be a person of broad basic education and catholicity of tastes based upon wide knowledge. We need not press the point that a wider interest in preventive medicine is one of the essential requirements of the day, but if the physician is to exercise this function effectively he must be a person of very broad culture and have at his disposal a vast amount of fundamental knowledge. These things are not to be obtained in a brief period of time, and if we are inclined to be critical of the increasing age at which students enter upon the active practice of medicine, our criticism may be sobered by facing the complexity of the problems with which the modern physician must deal and the improbability that stable judgment can be acquired by any cursory survey of the field. There has never been a time when wisdom based upon knowledge was more important to the practicing physician. This does not mean that there are no limits to the time which may wisely be spent upon medical education, but it does mean that he who must grasp the fundamental implications of most of the sciences should bring to it a trained mind, and that such intellectual preparation requires time for its development. The most cursory survey of the graduates of the medical schools in the last decade shows that a steadily increasing number of them have completed an undergraduate curriculum before entering upon their medical education. If with this be combined the group taking the so-called "combined course," which allows the inclusion of one year in the medical school toward a degree of Bachelor of Science, we shall find that a very handsome proportion of the medical graduates of today are in this group. Mere exposure to collegiate education is no guarantee of wisdom, but, other things being equal, the soundest medical practitioner will be obtained from the group which has had this opportunity. To this premedical preparation must be added not only the four years now required for the medical course but a period of at least one or even two years of hospital experience before entering upon general practice. This means that something approaching ten years must be spent after graduation from high school, or its equivalent, before the modern physician is equipped to enter practice. Those who would hold themselves out as specialists in any field must have a much longer preparation, and, though this has not yet been made the subject of accepted rules, something like five years after obtaining a medical degree should elapse before the medical student may be judged to be equipped as a finished specialist.

Let us next turn for a moment to the physical equipment which the modern physician must have at his disposal if he is to offer to his patients a really first-class article in diagnosis and treatment. Obviously he must be in a position to command the services of well-equipped laboratories where the problems of pathology, bacteriology, and chemistry can be promptly handled. He will have need of X ray apparatus for accurate judgments in many fields. If his practice is in urban neighborhoods, he can presumably use the equipment of a hospital with which he is, or should be, associated for such work. If his practice lie in the smaller places, he may have to supply himself with considerable laboratory equipment, and either alone, or with some colleague, employ technical assistance in this field. It is idle to attempt to enumerate what he must have because this will vary within the broadest limits, according to his particular situation, but it may be dogmatically asserted that these aids to diagnosis must be available and used. If they are not to be had at the hospital or at some commercial laboratory, then he will have to equip himself accordingly. At the very least he will have to have his stethoscope, his instruments for obtaining specimens of blood, his instrument for recording blood pressure, instruments for making nasal, rectal, and vaginal examinations, some apparatus for the treatment of fractures, and some instruments for minor surgical procedures. It is possibly not too much to suggest that he should have an electrically lighted ophthalmoscope, otoscope, and laryngoscope. Certain it is that if he is not equipped to use these instruments of precision he must be prepared to ask the assistance of those who are. In addition to this his automobile will cost him a tidy sum of money, and his telephone must have someone near it twenty-four hours a day. He will probably require the services of at least one woman, exercising some of the functions of a technician, a nurse, and a secretary. All of these things constitute an overhead with which his predecessor was not bothered, but which today will cut into his gross income to an amount running from 40 per cent upward. If he be a specialist, his equipment must be far more elaborate and much more expensive, and modern surveys tend to show that the overhead expenses of the modern specialist unattached to a group will eat up something like 60 per cent of his income.

II
MODERN MEDICAL DIAGNOSIS AND ITS REQUIREMENTS

No argument will be necessary in support of the dogmatic assertion that accurate diagnosis is the foundation of any sound plan for the care and oversight of health. It will also be obvious that at any given time in the progress of civilization those charged with the business of medical diagnosis should be prepared to bring to their task any or all of the scientific developments which have been proved important in supplying accurate data and in narrowing the field of guesswork. Much as we may admire the qualities and abilities of the family physician of forty years ago, we are bound to admit that many of his opinions were based upon inferences unsupported by accurate data and verging upon guesswork, enormously colored by diagnostic acumen resulting from his particular experience. That he was required to act upon such incomplete premises was due to the fact that science was, relatively speaking, in its infancy, and the facts which might have placed his opinions upon a secure basis were unobtainable. The extraordinary growth of scientific knowledge in the last thirty years has entirely reversed this situation. He, who today holds himself out to the community as a practitioner of medicine, or surgery, and bases his opinions upon guesswork when they might be based upon data scientifically accurate, or at least approaching scientific accuracy, is guilty of offering to his patients a shoddy article and narrowly avoids, if he avoids at all, the charge of quackery.

Diagnosis is no longer a simple business, but a highly complicated one. Under most conditions an opinion of considerable accuracy can be reached if the scientific aids to diagnosis are available and are used. For their availability the physician cannot always be held responsible, since many of them may require establishments and equipment quite beyond the reach of the individual physician. To this extent the public must bear the blame if such equipment is not available, and to that extent cannot charge negligence to the physician.

On the other hand, where such aids to diagnosis are available, and these today must include the skillful use of consultants in many fields, the physician can no longer hide behind "the cloak of mystery" and can no longer defend himself for an inaccurate diagnosis if he has not availed himself of all the methods which might have assisted his opinion. Commonly enough, average public opinion will require the application of many of the aids of science, but this is a very unsound and risky control upon the situation, since it is notorious that the public having obtained a half truth jumps to a conclusion and insists upon having various methods applied which in fact are neither desirable nor necessary under the particular existing circumstances. As an example may be noted the frequency with which patients now demand extensive X ray studies which are quite unnecessary for the particular situation and which serve no purpose other than that of increasing the expense. Here, as in many of the debatable fields in regard to the adjustment of modern medicine to the community, public opinion is necessarily uninformed, inaccurate, and prone to jump to conclusions. The public must ultimately come to realize that it is dependent for decisions of this character upon its experts in the medical field, and that public responsibility begins and ends with the insistence that the experts shall be informed, open-minded, and disinterested. Many of the most tragic blunders which have overtaken the public in its attempt to protect itself against disease have come about as the result of uninformed inexpert lay opinion attempting to deal with highly complicated technical questions and failing to take advantage of the presence in the community of capable experts upon whose opinion it might have relied.

Having laid down these general principles in regard to the atmosphere surrounding modern medical diagnosis, it is proper to point out briefly the extent and complication of available methods and the necessity that they shall be not only available but in fact be applied to the individual. Physical examination of forty years ago, as already pointed out, was a pretty sketchy and incomplete business, and very frequently failed to develop essential facts not then within the scope of the methods. With modern methods physical examination inevitably requires time and cannot safely be carried out in a hurried manner. The physician must at the outset take a detailed and complete history, which in view of his broader knowledge of the foundations of medicine will be a much more time-consuming process than that which was required of his predecessor. The time-honored method of generally surveying the patient and applying the tests of the senses is still required in order to give a certain roundness, and one might almost say humanity, to the procedure. This having been done, however, under average conditions the behavior of the circulation as shown by blood pressure should be determined, and routine examinations requiring capable laboratory technic must be made of the urine, the blood, and possibly of the sputum. Under a good many conditions X ray examination of the chest, and perhaps elsewhere, will be required. Under some conditions studies of metabolism will be indicated, and frequently tests of blood serum, particularly to determine the presence or absence of syphilis, should be regarded as a proper routine. Under many conditions bacteriological examinations of cultures from the throat, such other studies of the blood as the Widal reaction, and complicated chemical investigations throwing light upon the condition of kidney function may be indicated. In disease of the cardiovascular system X rays of the chest to determine the size and position of the heart, and perhaps the making of an electrocardiogram may be indicated. In disease in any portion of the intestinal tract, expert X ray examinations are often necessary. In the presence of injury, X ray examination becomes essential. It may be noted that at this point legal opinion has intruded itself into the field, the courts having repeatedly held that in the event of injury which may have produced a fracture, the failure to obtain X ray studies before treatment may constitute negligence on the part of the physician. In this case public opinion acting through another set of experts, often quite inept in the field, has to some extent cut the ground from under the physician and estopped him from exercising his expert judgment.

Should the question of disease of the urinary apparatus be at issue, quite complicated examinations—including at times searching bacteriologic tests, X ray examinations, chemical examinations of the blood and urine, and even the more complicated examinations of the urinary tract with cystoscope and ureter catheter—may be indicated. It would serve no useful purpose at this time to do more than indicate the breadth of the field of modern diagnosis and the fact that the physician is rarely in a position to postulate at the beginning of his examination that any particular line of investigation may not be required. Quite obviously, the physician acting in the capacity of the general practitioner must have at his disposal, in one way or another, all of these methods of study. It becomes a matter of opinion precisely at what point he will think it desirable to summon to his assistance another physician or physicians with special knowledge in their various fields. Consequently, it will at once be obvious that if the general practitioner is estopped for any reason—whether financial, environmental, or economic—from obtaining the services of required specialists, to that extent the whole machinery of modern medical diagnosis falls to the ground and the opinion of the physician retrogrades toward that given by his predecessors a generation ago.

In much modern discussion of the complicated question of adjusting medical service to modern conditions the phrase "the family physician" appears. From the trend of these discussions one is tempted to conclude that the phrase is used without careful consideration of the fact that at the beginning of the century it inevitably carried a very different connotation from that which is possible today. As previously pointed out, the physician of thirty or forty years ago as a rule practiced in a much smaller community and dealt with a much more stable population. In that day he could be in fact the physician of the family. Today this possibility has been severely curtailed. As will be subsequently pointed out, physicians today are practicing much more largely in the centers of population. The growth of hospitals, the development of specialization, and, perhaps most important, the increasing mobility of the population have radically altered this situation. The family doctor of the last century was a phenomenon suited to the social, economic, and scientific environment of the day. Under modern conditions he must be a very different type of person. His possibilities of profound personal knowledge of heredity and environment have largely disappeared. The possibility of his being in touch with a whole family is substantially at an end, many of the opinions which he quite light-heartedly expressed two generations ago could not now be accepted as satisfactory, and his whole approach to his patient has been extensively altered. It is better to revise our phrase to suit the altered facts, and to allow the dominating figure of the family physician to stand for all time in the nitch which he created for himself. Let us accept a more satisfactory successor in the form of the general practitioner who graduates by various steps into the modern internist, whose greatest single contribution to the community is in accurate diagnosis based upon thorough study and the proper assignment of patients to the care of whatever specialist may be indicated. It is perhaps worthwhile to reiterate the fact that the general practitioner of today must be a very different person, both in his training and in his actual association with patients, from his predecessor of forty years ago. Mere age and experience, though of primary importance in fitting scientific data to the individual, can no longer be substituted for facts obtained through the application of scientific method. It is today commonly true that the relatively recent graduate equipped to use modern diagnostic methods and with a satisfactory background of hospital experience is a safer adviser than his senior colleague approaching three score years whose education never included a knowledge of modern science, and who, in the turmoil of active practice, has been unable to keep himself reasonably abreast of the times. From the point of view of the aspiring young physician, his own position today is at marked advantage as compared with that which he would have had to face at the beginning of the century. The advantage of the senior practitioner of today lies largely in his extended knowledge of those considerable regions of human behavior which have not yet come accurately within the view of science.

Another point about which there is today much misapprehension is in regard to the extent and reasons for specialization in the field of medicine. For instance, one frequently sees it stated both in the medical and in the lay press that there are today too many specialists. Whether or not this statement is true depends entirely upon one's definition of a specialist. If one defines as a specialist all those who allege themselves to be expert in some particular field of medicine or surgery, then the statement may be true but, if on the contrary, one defines a specialist as one who has by prolonged study and experience equipped himself as an expert in some particular field, then I think the statement is violently untrue. It is my own well-considered opinion that at the present time there is not in the United States any excess of specialists, properly so-called.

Specialization has, in the first place, limited the field of endeavor. The physician has been enabled to keep more thoroughly abreast of the rapidly changing knowledge applicable to his particular field. Today it is probably possible for the specialist, if he properly organizes his work, to have at least a reasonable knowledge of the additions to ascertained fact and the methods of study and treatment available in his field. That all specialists do in fact keep abreast of knowledge is not here asserted.

Another important reason for specialization is that it provides a group of people who are in a position to apprehend the problems and the limitations of special knowledge in the field. It is to them, therefore, that the world looks in all branches for the investigation tending to the advancement of knowledge. They are most likely to be in a position to study the possibilities of utilizing new discoveries in various fields of science for application to the practice of medicine. That specialization has contributed to the extension of knowledge must be obvious, and this constitutes one of its most important claims to approval. It is becoming evident that there is a strong tendency on the part of the younger men entering the practice of medicine to so shape their plans as to tend toward specialization. A variety of reasons for this tendency have been assigned. A great deal of criticism, some of it probably justified, has been leveled at the heads of the medical educators, it being alleged that they have tended to stress the scientific aspects of the practice of medicine to the neglect of the human side. In the jargon of the trade, they have overweighed the science and undervalued the art of medical practice. Much of this criticism appears ill-considered, since it must be obvious that the business of the medical school is to place at the disposal of the student that scientific knowledge which is certainly basic in medical practice. It must further familiarize him with the scientific method of approach to medical problems. It is, of course, highly desirable that medical education should bring the student into contact with a very large number of human beings in all aspects of health and disease. On the other hand, no one who has been closely allied with medical education can overlook the very grave difficulties of putting this into practice. Even though the length of the medical course has been progressively extended from three to five or even six years—if one includes the hospital period—time and requirement for protection of the patients with which the medical student may have contact will severely limit the possibilities of placing him in the finished relation of patient and physician. It is safe to assert that the modern medical student is not exposed to too much contact with science, though it is certainly true that the extent to which his contact with patients can be extended should be increased by every possible method.

Certain economic aspects of specialization have had their day in court, it being somewhat light-heartedly said that the tendency of the rising generation of physicians to specialize is due to the fact that they see in the work of the specialist an easier method of earning a handsome income and a life freed from the constant interferences and worries of general practice. That some such vagrant thought may flit through the mind of the medical student perhaps convicts him of nothing more serious than being a normal human being. On the other hand, sufficient weight has not been given to a very different aspect of this question. The modern medical student in his contact with fundamental science and in his hospital experience, which today, to some extent, involve a period of four, or even five years, cannot avoid being impressed by the staggering amount of accurate knowledge required of the general practitioner if he is to offer to his patients a really first-class article of service. The boldest may well take pause in the face of such responsibilities. He sees without difficulty that by narrowing his field he stands at least some chance of being able capably to grasp it. He is impressed by the fact that in the hurry and turmoil of general practice many tragic errors occur, and he quite humanly hesitates to weight his conscience with the probability that in trying to grasp the whole field he may fail to master it in a fashion sufficiently comprehensive to enable him to live comfortably and at peace with his conscience. This aspect of specialization will deserve more serious consideration if we propose to continue the present plan of medical service. At the present time the more or less isolated general practitioner is under a strain which may well stagger anyone who contemplates assuming it. He must often practice his profession without prompt and effective access to modern diagnostic methods. He must frequently decide problems which are possibly within the realm of the specialist, and he must salve his conscience for errors of omission or commission with the realization that the organization of medical service permits him to do no better. Unless we propose to do something to relieve the burden of the general practitioner not working in considerable centers of population, we must be charitable to those who are unwilling at the outset to face such terrifying possibilities.

It remains to note briefly the social and economic changes which have occurred during this period with their inevitable effect upon the practice of medicine. A very important item has been the striking and progressive shift of population toward the cities. In 1890 the urban population of the United States was 22,298,359, while the rural population, defined as those living in incorporated places of less than 2,500 or in other rural territory, amounted to 40,649,-355.[1] In 1930 the urban population was 68,954,823, the rural population, 53,820,223. In this shift some other striking figures occur. In 1890 there lived, in cities of a million or over, 3,662,115, while in 1930 there lived, in such places, 15,064,555. The shift is even more striking in cities of 500,000 to a million. Thus in 1890 there were in these cities 806,343, while in 1930 there were 5,763,987—an increase of something like seven times. As compared with this may be taken the shift of population in cities of 2,500 to 5,000; in 1890 there were 2,506,827; in 1930, 4,717,590—considerably less than double the number. In general, it may be noted that while the rural population had increased some thirteen million, the urban population had increased from twenty-two million to sixty-eight million—more than three times as rapidly. Such a shift was bound to influence profoundly the status of the physician, for while in 1890 nearly two-thirds of the population lived in rural territory, in 1930 only about two-fifths lived there. This alone would importantly alter the status of the family physician who, as already pointed out, was probably at the height of his development at about the earlier period.

The movement to the cities, and particularly to the larger cities, obviously includes an increased rapidity of movement in general, and thus introduces into the population with which the general practitioner must deal a double element of unrest. In the first place there are a large number of newcomers continually arriving in the cities, and in the second place the movement of the population in connection with great industries from one industrial center to another is probably much increased. I shall deal in another chapter with the question of the shift of medical population during this period. It will be sufficient at the present time to point out that the movement of physicians from the country to the cities has not only kept abreast with the movement of the population, but has largely exceeded it. This fact should obviously be related in any discussion to the increase in specialization already referred to.

The changes which have taken place in transportation during the period are little short of revolutionary. The spread of railroad transportation went on rapidly and steadily, and reached a level which at the present time appears to be importantly in excess of modern requirements. The appearance of the automobile, followed by the building of hard surfaced roads, enormously reduced distance insofar as it is a factor in the mobility of population and in the radius over which a physician can distribute his services efficiently. In the last decade the increase in airplane transportation has become a very real factor in both of these fields, and it is today possible to supply consultants of first-class calibre to even the most out-of-the-way districts. By the same token it has become possible to transport ill or injured patients from localities where they cannot receive effective care to large centers of population and to transport injured men from the wilderness to civilization in a relatively few hours. Inseparable from this is the almost universal extension of telephone and telegraph which now makes it possible for physician and patient to communicate with each other and often to settle important problems over distances running up to some thousands of miles. Even the lowly gas station will accept telegraph messages presented by the light-hearted automobilist. With the development of wireless it has even become possible to give medical advice to vessels in mid-ocean.

All of these factors have contributed to extend physically the sphere of usefulness of the physician and to diminish the possibility of isolation, whether of the individual or the community. It has been of assistance in enabling the physician in a relatively isolated community to obtain the assistance of scientific methods and of his more specialized brethren when such requirements appeared. It is not, however, clear that these possibilities have been utilized to the fullest possible extent. Though time and space have been importantly contracted, economic considerations not rarely operate as a considerable limitation of the extent to which advantage is taken of that state of affairs. It does, however, render possible, at least in theory, the setting up of medical establishments which would offer complete medical service over an area altogether wider than has been possible at any previous period.

Only a cursory glance can be given to the changes taking place in industry during the same period. Though industry grew, the "trust" flourished, and "big business" appeared during this period, the largest single stimulus to development and change in industry was probably the result of the War. Here, under the pressure of necessity, was laid the basis of modern quantity production, a method which has apparently proceeded at a rate somewhat in advance of our ability to adjust ourselves or digest intellectually and morally its implications. As it concerns the practice of medicine, some very important developments have taken place. It was during this period that careful scientific study has been given to the development in industry of various diseases from conditions directly related thereto. It was also during this period that increasing and effective attention has been given to the avoidance of injury and to prompt and skillful management when it occurs. This has given rise to the development of what today amounts almost to a specialty, the care of industrial disease. This involves knowledge and familiarity with conditions not commonly seen by the general practitioner, and is coming to be a branch of special practice which may be expected to develop further as time goes on. It has also given rise to the development by industry of its own medical and even hospital establishments. This has come about largely as the result of increased competition under the pressure of which it has become clear that industry can neither afford to employ physically unsound people, nor can it afford to allow the ailments which develop either on account of or incidental to employment to be managed in anything short of an effective manner. This has led to a considerable extension of the preliminary medical examination of employees and has in some cases been carried to the point of requiring a periodic physical examination. It has also resulted in the setting up of emergency establishments by industry for the immediate care of the injured and also to elaborate medical establishments which at times include the offering to the employees and even to their families of complete medical care, sometimes free of charge, and sometimes for a modest contribution from wages. A fuller discussion of the developments of industrial medicine will be found in a later chapter.

It is further important to note a change which has apparently taken place in the view which industry is taking of its relation to society. Up to about the beginning of the century many or most of the great industrial ventures of the country were largely the work of single individuals of great courage and intellectual ability. One need only point to the development of the railroads, to the development of the oil industry, to the development of the coal and the iron industries, to call to mind great individuals from whose efforts these industries grew to great power and influence. It is not so many years since the unexpected death of one of these great "magnates" would have shaken seriously the financial structure of the country, and one can remember the closing of stock exchanges on such occasions, not apparently from any profound reverence for the character of the late lamented. This situation has been very importantly altered during the last two decades, and it is probably safe to assert that there is today no individual short of the President of the United States whose sudden death would seriously disturb the financial structure of the country. This is not due to the fact that great intellectual capacity is not being brought to the service of industry, but to the fact that the responsibility for the conduct of these great businesses is, under modern methods, distributed among several individuals so that a group and not a single person controls their destinies. Whether this change has come about as a result or is the chief cause, the fact appears clear that today industry is more conscious of and sensitive to its social obligations than at any previous period. It appears to me that there is very clear evidence of the development in business of a code of ethics which at certain levels bids fair to put the business executive on a basis properly called professional. This has the effect of bringing him closely into contact with the other professional groups of the Church, the Law, and Medicine, and one is likely to find in all these groups today people of quite similar intellectual interest. It is probably not an accident that during this period there have sprung up in the educational world schools of business administration whose ideals and practices are approaching those of the other professional schools under similar auspices. That the effect of such schools will be to alter the social outlook of those who will in the future direct industrial enterprises is perhaps a reasonable assumption. This may become of prime importance in any consideration of the extent to which medical service should be further socialized. In any plan which we may entertain for the adjustment of medical service to modern economic conditions we shall be well advised to bear in mind this obvious shift in the social and moral control of industry.

During this same period and to some extent running parallel with the changes in industry above noted has come a change in the relation of the farmer to society. During the time when there was much unoccupied land, and the area devoted to agriculture was still relatively small in relation to its ultimate possibility, the farmer, at least to some extent and certainly sufficiently to influence very much the character of rural practice, was a person whose primary intent was to live on the land, raising enough for the support of his family and a moderate surplus for sale. Beginning at a time quite definitely before that which we have selected as characteristic of the changes in medical practice, this situation insensibly changed and the farmer became progressively less self-sufficient and moved steadily toward the capitalist class. More and more the farmer became engaged in a business which required outside financing. Mortgages on land and for the purchase of equipment became increasingly common. Even in the middle Nineties the effect of this change was very evident, and was accentuated by the financial difficulties of 1893. This, however, in no way altered the inevitable development and the World

War, with its accompanying high prices for farm products, pushed the farmer further into the capitalist class. In the best of times very handsome incomes were earned upon the investment, and a good many farmers found the venture sufficiently profitable so that with advancing years they could retire and move into the larger towns or even abandon the venture entirely and move to other parts of the country. As time went on, however, the difficulties of operating the farm on a capitalistic basis became increasingly evident, and had two effects bearing upon the practice of medicine. In the first place it tended to the immense increase in the size of the farms with a relative diminution in the number of people employed. With the extensive introduction of farm machinery both the relative and, at times, even the absolute number of people required to handle the crops diminished. In the second place, the necessity for borrowed capital often rendered the financial situation of the farmer increasingly precarious, and undoubtedly part of the migration from country to city was of this origin, though of course the tremendous growth of industry was the chief magnet. But it affected the practice of medicine not only in diminishing the number of people in rural communities, but in making the collection of reasonable fees increasingly uncertain, and, during the last half decade, precarious.

There finally remains for us to consider at this time the phenomenal growth in the number, size, and use of hospitals. This is a development of such importance as to require separate consideration, but it will be worthwhile at this time to recall that until about the beginning of the present century the use of hospitals was, relatively speaking, uncommon as compared with the present day, and that most of the hospital patients were either mentally abnormal or indigent. The forces leading to the increased use of hospitals were partly economic and partly social. With the revolution in surgery which followed the acceptance of the doctrines of Pasteur and Lister in regard to the control of infection, hospitals became relatively safe places, and, with the enormous increase in the amount of surgical treatment much of which could only be carried out to the best advantage in hospital surroundings, the importance of hospital care became increasingly evident. On the social side, it became more and more difficult to carry out the necessary precautions in private houses. In the early part of this century, the choice presented to an individual faced with a surgical operation was whether or not it was cheaper to turn his house into a hospital or temporarily to lease a portion of a hospital for the purpose. During this same period hospital construction became much more perfect, and the development of nursing service was rapid. It thus became increasingly evident that for severe illness or surgical operation the surroundings of the hospital were not only more conducive to recovery, but less disturbing to the economic and social environment of the patient. A part in the transition was also played by the increasing complexity of medical diagnosis and treatment, both of which required equipment not to be had except in hospital surroundings, or only at almost prohibitive expense. As evidence of the trend of the times, the growth and development of hospital social service is important. Medical social service had its origin in the evidence that in large hospitals and particularly in those intended largely for indigent or partly indigent patients there was grave danger of the development of two evils. One was that in the attempt on the part of the physician to give as much service as possible, he might quite fail to make sufficiently intimate contact with the patient to convey to him accurately his opinions and plans for treatment. The other grew out of the increasing complication of medical care and the growth of methods of treatment other than the giving of medicine. Obviously, in crowded hospital practice the time of the physician could be best spent in those fields for which he was primarily best equipped—namely, in diagnosis and in the parts of treatment requiring his special service. But, there remained a very large amount of treatment which required detailed explanation to the patient so that he might understand the underlying causes. Particularly where methods such as changes in habits of life, changes of diet, and the prolonged use of various types of physical therapy were concerned, it was essential that the social and economic conditions of the patient should be clearly understood and that the treatment should be adapted to the possibilities, and not based upon ideal conditions having no real existence. Undoubtedly, the development and spread of social service has helped the hospitals to avoid to some extent the charge of an impersonal relation and an ineffective carrying out of treatment.

III

OUR MEDICAL RESOURCES

No discussion of the present or future condition of medical practice can proceed far without a certain basic understanding of the material which the community has at its disposal for dealing with this problem. Obviously, of this material, the supply and distribution of physicians, hospitals, and nurses will form a major factor.

NUMBER OF PHYSICIANS

The number of physicians in June, 1932, was approximately 156,440, giving a ratio to population of about one physician to every 780 persons.[1] It is interesting to note that the number of physicians per capita of population has always been higher in this country than in other countries. An accurate figure probably cannot be obtained, as the source of information is the United States Census, which prior to 1910 drew no distinction between physicians and other healers, and prior to 1920 did not differentiate between physicians and osteopaths. However, allowing for this margin of error, it appears that in 1850 there was one physician to every 569, that in 1890 there was one physician to every 601, that in 1920 there was one physician to every 642 and that in 1932 there was one physician to every 780.[2] Thus, the proportion of physicians has been slowly but steadily falling, and this appears to be true, not only for the United States as a whole, but for most of its subdivisions. On the other hand, there is a very striking difference in the ratio of physicians to population in different sections of the country. In the West North Central states there was, in 1920, one physician to every 587 of the population, in the Pacific states one physician to every 410, while in the South Atlantic states there was one physician to every 910.[3] A still more striking figure is a recent one showing that California has one physician to 483 people, while North and South Carolina have one to about 1,430.[4] It is interesting to compare these figures with the ratio of physicians to population in other countries.

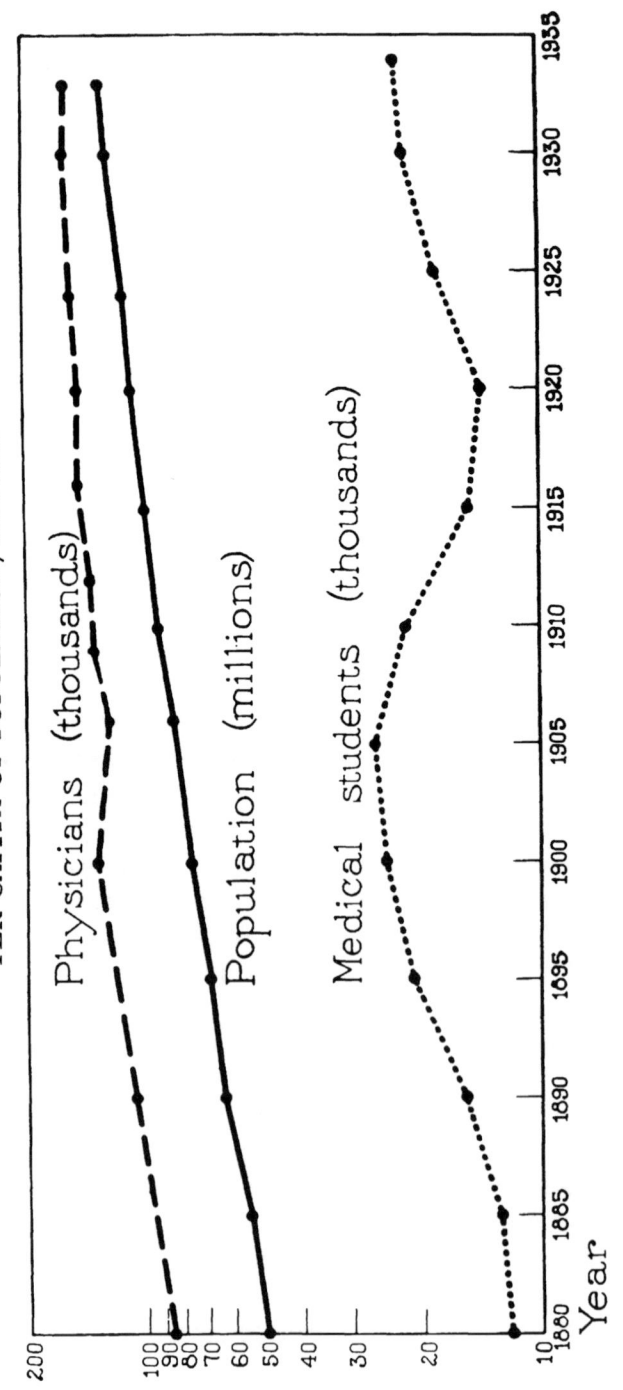

PHYSICIANS, MEDICAL STUDENTS, AND TOTAL POPULATION, 1880-1935

(Statistical summary of data used in the preparation of the chart on the opposite page.)

YEAR	PHYSICIANS	MEDICAL STUDENTS	TOTAL POPULATION
1880	85,671 [a]	12,000 [a]	50,155,783 [g]
1885		12,800 [a]	55,000,000 [a]
1890	104,805 [a]	15,500 [a]	62,947,714 [g]
1895		20,900 [a]	69,000,000 [a]
1900	132,002 [a]	24,500 [a]	75,994,575 [g]
1905		26,147 [d]	
1906	122,028 [b]		83,000,000 [a]
1909	134,402 [h]		
1910		21,800 [a]	91,972,266 [g]
1912	137,199 [h]		
1915		15,200 [a]	99,000,000 [a]
1916	145,241 [b]		
1920	145,404 [h]	13,798 [d]	105,710,620 [g]
1924	147,010 [h]		111,000,000 [a]
1925		18,200 [d]	
1930	156,406 [f]	21,597 [d]	122,775,046 [g]
1933	154,495 [e]		125,692,606 [a]
1934		22,799 [d]	

[a] Mayers and Harrison, The Distribution of Physicians in the United States, New York, General Medical Board, 1924, p. 162. [b] Ibid., p. 159. [c] Ibid., p. 160.
[d] "Medical Education in the United States and Canada," Journal of the American Medical Association, Vol. 103, August 25, 1934, p. 574. [e] Ibid., p. 577. [f] Ibid., p. 578.
[g] Abstract of the Fifteenth Census of the United States, 1930, p. 9. [h] American Medical Directory, 1934, p. 16.

Thus in England and Wales the ratio is one to 1,490, in Germany, one to 1,560, in France, one to 1,690, and in the Scandinavian countries—Denmark, Norway, and Sweden—one to 2,156. Now, on the face of it, the casual observer might conclude that as compared with the rest of the civilized world, these United States had too many doctors. Nevertheless, some ten years ago there arose a very considerable outcry, most noticeable in the medical journals, but permeating the lay press, to the effect that medical service in the United States was breaking down, and that there were considerable areas where medical service was not available. Obviously, the problem is not one of total number of physicians, nor even of the number of physicians in any section or state in the country, but rather one of the distribution of these physicians so that their services are available. The tendency of the population to move from rural to urban areas, already noted, has affected the distribution of physicians very profoundly. Thus, in 1906, cities of over 25,000 inhabitants included 28 per cent of the population and 40 per cent of the physicians of the country. In 1923, such cities contained 37 per cent of the population and over 50 per cent of the physicians.[5] A study of the tendencies of recent graduates in medicine shows that they are quite as much affected as the figure for the whole group would show. A study of the distribution of graduates of the classes of 1920 and 1925 shows that 31.6 per cent of each group settled in cities of over 500,000—containing only 17 per cent of the population—and that, respectively, 18.1 per cent and 20.8 per cent settled in cities of from 100,000 to 500,000, containing 12.6 per cent of the population. Thus, it is clear that of the recent graduates over 50 per cent settled in cities of 100,000 or over, containing only 29.6 per cent of the population, whereas 47.8 per cent settled in cities under 100,000, containing 70.4 per cent of the population.[6] If, therefore, it appears that the total number of physicians in the country is adequate, it obviously follows that the profession in the cities of 100,000 or over is tremendously overcrowded. As evidence of this may be taken the ratio of physicians to population in towns and cities of various size in 1906 and 1923. Thus in cities of 100,000 or more, the ratio of physicians to population in 1906 was one to 488; and in 1923, one to 544. In contrast to this, the ratio of physicians in towns having a population of from 1,000 to 2,500 was in 1906 one to 590; and in 1923, one to 910.[7] In general it may be said that the falling off in the number of physicians per capita has been most rapid in the places having less than 5,000 inhabitants.

There is another fact which has appeared in the study of this question; namely, the average age of physicians in the smaller towns is increasing as compared with the larger cities. This, of course, is only another way of saying that the younger men are not going to the smaller places and that the physicians resident there have the habit common to mankind of growing older—a disease for which there is as yet no discovered cure.

Causes of Changing Distribution

Obviously, a part of the changing distribution of physicians is nothing but a reflection of the general shift of population, but, as has been shown above, the shift in physicians has clearly exceeded the shift in population and there is no evidence as yet that the tendency is diminishing. There must, therefore, be factors other than those causing the general shift of population which are here involved. Perhaps the largest single factor arises from the altered condition of medical practice previously discussed. Insofar as the most satisfactory type of modern medical practice requires the proximity of laboratories and other complicated equipment, to precisely that extent will the practice of medicine in the smaller places become less and less satisfactory. Another aspect of the same question is the very steady increase in specialization, since the specialist obviously cannot survive except in centers of population where some division of practice can be satisfactorily carried out. Another factor which has certainly operated to alter the ratio is the development of means of transportation. At an earlier day a distance of ten miles or more was a serious, or even prohibitive, distance at which to seek medical advice. Today, in many parts of the country with improved roads and at many seasons even without them, the introduction of the automobile has made ten miles as nothing. This means that patients, who, at an earlier day were practically required by circumstances to consult the physician in the village, not only can but do light-heartedly crank up their automobile and buzz by his door to the larger town where they have, or think they have, the possibility of a greater range of medical opinion. There is much testimony tending to show that the physician in the small village of 1,000 inhabitants or less will today starve to death, though there are abundant people within a reasonable radius who at a former time would have consulted him. It has been estimated that somewhere between 1,000 and 1,200 people are necessary to the support of a physician, and it is implicit in this estimate that these people will in fact utilize his services and not utilize their automobiles to seek service at a greater distance.

A great variety of other reasons have been put forward as the cause for the disappearance of physicians in rural areas. For instance, it has been argued that the length of the present medical course, which during the period under consideration has been extended from three to five or six years, has thrown upon the medical student an expense which requires him when he enters practice to demand an income higher than that which his predecessor required. In this argument the increased length of training and the expense of the medical course may be taken together, since, though there has been an actual increase in the expense per year necessary to get good medical education, the chief item in the bill is the increased length of the course. Two points may be noted as tending to lessen the weight of this argument. If it be true—and there seems to be substantial evidence upon the point—that the physician in the rural districts cannot now earn a livelihood which will enable him to keep body and soul together, it makes very little difference whether the medical course has cost him $4,000.00 or $10,000.00, since in neither case can he look forward to an income which will enable him to live in reasonable economic comfort. The view that a shorter and less expensive course would influence recent graduates to settle in the smaller places does not seem to be compatible with the evidence of distribution of graduates from one of the large schools of chiropractic. Thus, a study of the distribution of over 2,000 graduates of one of the largest of these schools, which gives a course considerably shorter than that of medicine, shows that 90.2 per cent of the graduates located in communities of 50,000 or more. This is a very much higher proportion than that of recent medical graduates.[8]

As a matter of fact, there is experience elsewhere with the production of less completely trained or sub-standard physicians. Many European countries tried this system. Austria, in particular, during the nineteenth century had such courses for country doctors. They were at first only two years in length, but were extended in 1810 to three years. Various attempts to abolish this output of sub-standard practitioners were made, notably in 1848; but it was not until 1872 that the training of such physicians was definitely discontinued.[9]

It has also been alleged that the failure of recent graduates to settle in the smaller places is due to the faulty character of medical training. The argument runs somewhat as follows. Modern medical education requires of the student during his first two years an enormous amount of laboratory work in the fundamental sciences. During the latter part of his course he sees patients only in the hospital, and commonly with serious or unusual conditions. This is further accentuated by his intern or hospital experience where he is called upon to deal chiefly with those conditions which can only be handled satisfactorily under hospital conditions.

Though this leaves out of account the number of patients seen in the dispensary and out-patient department, it may be at once admitted that the training of the medical student does not, in fact, bring him in contact with the conditions of the general practice of medicine. That this should be held to be a satisfactory explanation of the trend of physicians to the cities, or that alteration of the medical curriculum is indicated, cannot, however, be admitted. It is not suggested that the physicians in general, and particularly in isolated practice, should be less familiar with serious conditions and with the scientific methods of diagnosis and treatment. In fact there will be general agreement with the dogmatic statement that the isolated physician must be a person of broader knowledge and wider capacity than the one who practices in a large community and who can obtain the help of complicated scientific methods and prompt assistance of his professional brethren. If it is desired to increase the capacity of the practitioner who must deal nearly single-handed with the problems of medicine, then a longer and more varied preliminary experience is clearly indicated.

The nub of this question is not whether there are more or less physicians in any given locality than there were thirty years ago, but whether or not medical service now available is the equal of that offered at the earlier period. On that point opinion will of necessity differ. It is certainly true that the improved methods of transportation have, for most of the smaller communities, made medical service more rather than less available. Thirty years ago the town or community hospital was largely nonexistent. At that period, to summon a physician from a distance of thirty, or even twenty, miles was hardly to be considered, except for the most serious conditions, and would have consumed the greater part of a day, or even more, of his time. Today the average physician in towns where there are plenty of hard surfaced roads, and where specialization has to a considerable extent occurred, thinks nothing of making two or three visits at fifteen to thirty miles from his office as a part of his ordinary routine. It is, of course, true that improvement in transportation has not made country roads passable at all seasons of the year. It is true that at certain periods towns may be completely isolated, though less so today than at any earlier period. Nevertheless, it may confidently be asserted that even with the important diminution in the number of physicians available in the rural districts medical service is today at least the equal of that offered at any earlier period. It should be borne in mind that the development of the telephone has added considerably to the area over which the influence of the physician can be exerted. For instance, a physician who years ago would have been entirely isolated can today by means of the telephone discuss his complicated problems with a colleague perhaps at a considerable distance, and, in this way, broaden his information in regard to the situation. Furthermore, it is now frequently possible for physicians even in relatively isolated communities to keep in closer contact with their patients by means of the telephone than was previously possible. This has the effect of enabling the physician to get early information in regard to the development of unexpected complications and to so plan his time as to see those patients most frequently who are in most need of his services. Thus, it may reasonably be doubted whether the rural population of this country has today at its disposal medical service in any respect inferior to that which it has enjoyed in the past.

When one comes to discussing the question of whether medical service to the rural community as supplied at the present time, or at any period in the past, would be judged adequate as measured by modern standards, the case is quite reversed. If we assume, for the moment, a conclusion which will be more thoroughly developed later —that adequate medical service at the present time requires that there shall be available to everybody reasonable access to modern methods of diagnosis and treatment—it may readily appear that there are very large groups in the community for whom such service is not available. But, it should also be remembered that the rural population has no monopoly of this lack of service. There are undoubtedly in the large cities today enormous numbers of people who for purely financial reasons are unable to get medical service which will match reasonable modern requirements.

Supply and Training of Medical Graduates

During the last fifty years the number of medical schools in the United States has varied within very wide limits. In 1880 there were 100 medical schools having 11,826 students and 3,241 graduates of that year. During the next twenty years the number of schools rose rapidly so that by 1900 there were 160 schools with 25,171 students and 5,214 graduates of that year. The high point was reached in 1906 with 162 schools.[10] Many of these schools were purely commercial ventures. Some of them might properly be classified as diploma mills, and many of them were organized by groups of physicians with the scarcely veiled intention of providing, through their students, feeders for their practice as consultants. The unsatisfactory character of this situation was brought sharply to public attention by the publication by the Carnegie Foundation for Advancement of Teaching of the book by Mr. Abraham Flexner entitled "Medical Education in the United States and Canada." This report clearly established the fact that much of the medical education then given in the country was on an unsatisfactory basis, and that the educational requirements prior to the study of medicine were insufficient to warrant a high grade of intellectual capacity in the student. The facts thus brought out led to action by the American Medical Association, through its Council on Medical Education, which resulted in a classification of schools, and consequent indirect pressure for improvement. The reaction following this report—and I think importantly due to the report—coupled with the wise activity of the American Medical Association and the Association of American Medical Colleges, brought very prompt results. Within the next ten years, the number of medical schools had decreased to 96, the students to 14,891, and the graduates to 3,536.[11]

Up to 1910 a relatively small percentage of the medical students had previous academic degrees. In that year 15 per cent had either the A.B. or the B.S. degree. Since that time the percentage has steadily increased until, in 1932, 71 per cent were holders of such degrees.[12] The diminution in number of schools continued up to 1929, when it reached its present number of 76.[13] Of this number, ten offer only the first two years of the medical courses, and their students must therefore take the latter part of the course elsewhere. There are at the present time 66 schools in the United States and 9 schools in Canada furnishing most of the medical graduates entering practice in the United States. The falling off of the number of students and graduates was, as has been shown, quite sharp at first; but, though the number of schools diminished, the number of graduates has increased progressively until in 1932 the 76 schools had 22,135 students and 4,936 graduates, the latter figure approaching that at the high point in 1904, 5,747.[14] See Graph 1, page 36.

At the present time all of these schools require at least two years of college work prior to admission, and as has been pointed out above, some 70 per cent of the students either hold a bachelor's degree or are on the so-called combined course which leads to the awarding of a B.S. degree at the conclusion of their first year in the medical school. It is thus clear that since 1910 the improvement in the academic requirements has been striking and progressive. For the average student at the present time the university preparation for the practice of medicine requires seven years. To this has been added by fifteen states, the District of Columbia, and Alaska, the requirement of a year's hospital training before the degree is awarded.[15] At the present time the medical course will average nearly eight years for most students. This change has had the effect of increasing the age at which medical graduates enter the practice of medicine. Quoting from the Final Report of the Commission on

Medical Education: "During recent years the average age at which medical students have graduated has been just under twenty-seven years. The median age is nearer twenty-six years."

There is also a certain number of physicians educated in foreign countries who come here and are licensed to practice by the various state examining boards. This number, of recent years, has not been very large. It was apparently at its height in 1925 when 610 physicians from other countries were licensed to practice. Of these, 292 came from Canada, so that the number from all other countries was relatively small. This number has diminished, and the figures for 1929 show a total of 278, of whom 149 came from Canada.[16]

In general terms, the number of well-trained graduates now being turned out in this country would seem sufficient to provide the necessary physicians, unless some very profound change in our system of medical practice should occur.

Growth and Development of Hospitals

No clear grasp of the medical facilities available, or likely to be available, for the care of illness can be obtained without some conception of the growth, development, distribution, and type of hospitals.

A pretty careful survey of the field in 1872 appeared to show that, at that time, there were in the United States 178 hospitals having a total capacity of 35,604 beds.[17] In 1900 there are said to have been about 1,000 hospitals, while in 1931 there were 6,613.[18] In 1920 there were one or more hospitals in only 44 per cent of the counties of the country, while in 1931, 70 per cent of the counties were so provided. Perhaps a little different slant on the rate of development and capacity may be had if we realize that "during the last twenty-two years, hospitals have been built and equipped at the rate of one sixty-nine bed hospital each day, including Sundays and holidays." [19] These hospitals are now admitting patients at the rate of fourteen patients per minute.

The hospitals of the country may be divided into groups according to their ownership. Thus, government hospitals, meaning all hospitals owned by units of the government and including the federal, state, county, and city hospitals, in 1931 numbered 1,816, had a bed capacity of 641,524, and admitted 1,833,078 patients. The non-government hospitals, including those owned by church organizations, fraternities, industry, corporations, and individuals, numbered 4,797, had a bed capacity of 332,591, and admitted 5,322,898.[20] From these figures it will at once appear that while the bed capacity of government-owned hospitals is nearly double that of the non-government hospitals, they admit during the year only about one-third as many patients. This is a reflection of the fact that the state hospitals are likely to be asked to care for many cases of chronic disease, and particularly those having mental and nervous disease. These patients have a notoriously long stay in the hospital, running often into a matter of years, and in this way more or less sterilize a large number of beds. It is interesting to note that the average bed occupancy is much higher in government-owned hospitals than in the other group. Thus, for all government-owned hospitals the average bed occupancy was 88.7 per cent, while for the non-government-owned hospitals it was 61.9 per cent. A still more striking contrast will be obtained if it is noted that the average bed occupancy in state hospitals, as distinguished from other types of government hospitals, was, during the years 1929, 1930, and 1931, about 94 per cent. This, again, reflects the large number of patients who are wards of the state for long periods of time. The extent to which the public has become accustomed to the use of hospitals is, perhaps, satisfactorily shown by the following comparison: In 1904 there were in the United States about 1,400,000 patients admitted to hospitals, while in 1931 there were about 12,000,000.[21] This by no means tells the whole story, since a very large number of patients who are not admitted to hospitals are yet consulting physicians at public clinics and dispensaries, and are in this sense hospital patients. "The number of clinics and dispensaries has risen from 150 in 1900 to almost 8,000 at present."[22] A somewhat different view may be had of the same development by a comparison between the number of outpatient departments of hospitals, which in 1921 amounted to 678 and in 1931 to 2,042.[23] As concerns the utilization of these outpatient departments, in 1921 there were 3,000,163 patients treated, while in 1931 there were 6,962,724. Evidently, during this period the patients had acquired more confidence in these organizations, for while in 1927, 6,750,388 patients made 13,804,566 visits—or an average of slightly over two visits per patient—in 1931, 6,962,724 patients made 23,431,382 visits—three and two-fifths visits.[24]

Parallel with this increasing use of hospitals by patients went, of course, an increasing use of hospitals by doctors. At a considerably earlier period the proportion of physicians having any form of regular affiliation with a hospital was relatively small, but increased steadily. By 1928, 90,903 physicians had some definite connection with a hospital, the great majority holding some type of visiting staff position. In 1931, 116,363 physicians had a similar relation.[25]

The Supply of Trained Nurses

A well-rounded health service will require physicians, nurses, and hospitals for its progressive development. Nursing is a relatively young profession in this country, and has, in fact, grown up chiefly during the forty years which we have here had under survey. Its development has importantly paralleled that of the hospitals.

In 1900 there were about 432 schools of nursing in the United States, in 1926 there were 2,155. In 1900 there were something less than 12,000 graduate nurses practicing in this country, in 1926 there were in the neighborhood of 180,000. It will be observed, therefore, that the increase in available trained nurses during the period of twenty-five years has been enormous. We may admit at once that at the earlier period the number of nurses available in the country was far below that urgently needed for medical service at that period. It is, I think, somewhat less certain that the number of nurses at the present time available does not at least approach the number which can properly be utilized.

In regard to the fields of work in which nurses are now engaged, something like 55 per cent of the nurses already graduated from hospitals enter the field of private practice. Of the remainder, some 23 per cent take positions in institutional work, and some 19 per cent are engaged in the broad field of public health nursing. This means, of course, that more than half of the nurses are engaged in free and open competition, and that they must meet the competition not only of their professional equals, but of everybody else who sees fit to call herself a nurse whether she is trained or not. Unfortunately, the public is not well equipped to distinguish a thoroughly trained graduate of a first-class school from a nurse with very insufficient training, or even none at all. Furthermore, there is no available method by which the group of thoroughly competent nurses can protect themselves, or be protected, against this sort of competition. It is, therefore, wise to recognize at the outset that those who elect the field of private duty nursing must stand a competition fierce and uncontrolled.

INCOME OF NURSES [26]

What income may nurses reasonably expect, having completed their training? Most of us, I think, who have not looked into the matter would be surprised at what appear to be carefully established facts. The median income of the private duty nurses in this country about 1926 was $1,297.00. This appears small in view of the fact that the average compensation at that period was $6.00 a day. It, of course, means that the private duty nurse is not regularly employed, and a fairly careful study appears to show that, what with considerable periods when they are out of work and such periods as they take for vacations, they do, in fact, work and earn their income in approximately seven months of the year. Out of this princely income must be taken such expenses as are necessary for living. If they have the good fortune to live at home, well and good. Otherwise a considerable slice of their income will be eaten up by the necessary requirements of board and lodging, for though a nurse may not be occupying her quarters more than half of the time, she will usually have to pay for them. As compared with this, the institutional nurse is better off. Her average median income is $2,000.00. Those engaged in public health service come between the two, and show a median income of about $1,685.00.

PRIVATE DUTY NURSING

It may next be interesting to inquire why such a large proportion of the nurses graduating from the schools seek private duty nursing, which on the face of the record is obviously overcrowded. The reasons are very human ones. They want freedom of action. They want liberty to pick and choose, to select the kind of nursing with which they are most familiar, and to work under the conditions to which they are best suited. They do not like to take cases in rural districts. They do not like to accept from the registry calls for any type of nursing work. They prefer to confine their work to certain fields, to work for certain physicians, and quite clearly they prefer to act as special nurses for patients in hospitals where they are surrounded by the conditions with which they are familiar. These reasons are wholly understandable, they are wholly human, but they are not wholly reasonable. If, as may properly be assumed, the average private duty nurse feels that her income is less than her ability entitles her to, this situation is the necessary and probable consequence of the fierce competition in which she is engaged. If she makes this choice, she must, for the present at least, face its implications.

INSTITUTIONAL NURSING

Those who are charged with the business of selecting candidates for institutional work report that, while they have many applicants for positions, a considerable proportion of them are less completely trained and less thoroughly competent than the positions properly require. It is, at least, suggested that if there were a larger supply of nurses thoroughly well-equipped for institutional work, more jobs would be available.

PUBLIC HEALTH NURSING

A very similar situation appears to exist in the field of public health nursing, where it is reported that there are five applicants for every job, but, chiefly because their training and experience is insufficient, many are not accepted.

IV

THE GENERAL PRACTICE OF MEDICINE

The right to practice medicine in the United States is based wholly upon licensure. In the regulation of medical practice throughout the world two principal methods are used: one, the principle of licensure by state authority, which forbids the practice of medicine by those not holding a license; and two, the principle of the establishment of a Register, a list upon which are placed the names of all those who have satisfied the requirements. Under the latter method other persons may practice medicine, but they are seriously handicapped in that they cannot perform certain official functions, such as the signing of death and birth certificates, and cannot make use of the courts to collect their fees. Curiously enough, although throughout the British Empire the method of registration is generally used, one of the earliest examples of licensure was the license issued to the Barbers of London in 1442 authorizing them to treat wounds, let blood, and draw teeth. In 1521 a charter was issued to the Royal College of Physicians in England, and later the Master Barbers Association became the Royal College of Surgeons.

It is important to appreciate at the outset that the purpose, whether of licensure or registration, is the protection of the public, and not the creation for practitioners of medicine of a preferred position. In the United States there was no accepted method and generally no method at all during Colonial times, and, prior to the development of medical schools, the practice of medicine was carried on by people who had obtained some training either by apprenticeship to physicians in the colonies or by study abroad. The first medical school was that of the University of Pennsylvania, founded in 1765. In 1772 New Jersey passed a law requiring licensing of the medical practitioners by two judges of the Supreme Court, with such assistance as they might require. In 1781 the Massachusetts Medical Society was chartered and, thereby, given power to examine and approve candidates for the practice of medicine. In the same year the New Hampshire Medical Society was chartered with similar powers. From 1825 onward, there grew up a miscellaneous assortment of alleged methods of medical practice—including Homeopathy, Thomsonianism, Eclecticism, and Botanics. This led to a tendency on the part of state legislatures, beginning in 1835, to take from the medical societies the power of approval, and to vest it in examining boards created by the states. This practice, however, was apparently not satisfactory, the number of physicians was below that desired, and in many states the laws creating the examining boards were repealed. At the time of the Civil War there was very little regulation of the practice of medicine, the creation of new states relatively inaccessible, and the shortage of practitioners probably being the cause. About 1870, however, there returned agitation for restrictive laws. Texas set up a licensing board in 1873, New York and Kentucky in 1874, and New Hampshire in 1875, and California and Vermont in 1876. By 1895 practically all the states had such boards.[1]

It will be seen that a reasonably uniform method of medical licensure has been in existence less than forty years, and, unlike most other countries of the world, the United States has no national system, the matter being left entirely in the hands of various states, with resulting differences of practice. Since the development of state boards of licensure by all of the states, the custom has grown up of licensing physicians by reciprocity in case they moved from one state to another. There is, of course, insistence that the requirements of the state in which the physician already has a license to practice shall be the equal of those in the state to which he desires to move. In general terms, the movement of physicians from one state to another has not been seriously impeded, but this is by no means universally true, and in certain instances there is serious interference with the free movement of physicians from one part of the country to another. This difficulty has been somewhat alleviated by the establishment in 1915 of the National Board of Medical Examiners, a voluntary organization having no governmental relation, but which conducts a series of three examinations: the first of which may be taken at the end of two years in the medical school; the second, at the end of four years; and the third, after the graduate has had at least one year of hospital experience. These examinations are severe and searching, more strict than those of most of the states. As a result, the graduates who have obtained a certificate from the National Board are now accepted by the licensing boards of forty-one states and three territories. The number of graduates taking this examination is, however, still small. In 1931, 419 certificates were issued, equal to about 9 per cent of the number of graduates of approved schools in 1930.[2]

The licenses granted to physicians are entirely general, authorize them to practice medicine and surgery, and do not assume any especial qualifications beyond those required of the general practitioner. In the earlier days this was obviously all that could be done, but the tremendous development of specialization, particularly in this country, has called attention to the fact that, as far as the public is concerned, anyone, whether with or without the requisite qualifications, may declare himself to be a specialist in any field, and confine his practice to any extent that he sees fit. On the other hand, there have developed inside of the profession various methods by which the qualifications of persons holding themselves out to be specialists in certain fields are reviewed and passed upon by the profession itself. Thus there has grown up the American College of Surgeons, and the American College of Physicians, each of which scrutinizes with considerable care the training of candidates for membership to the end that it shall appear that they have had a sufficient amount of postgraduate work to qualify them as experts and consultants in the respective fields of surgery and medicine. There have also been developed, by certain special medical groups, boards of examiners to pass upon the qualifications of those who desire their stamp of approval. The earliest of these was created by the American Society of Ophthalmologists, and, subsequently, similar boards have been created by the obstetricians, gynecologists, and others. It is thus evident that the medical profession is aware of the danger of unqualified specialists and has taken some steps to enable the public to ascertain, though with some difficulty, that a given physician has the requisite qualifications as a specialist.[3]

It will be remembered that in the nineteenth century there grew up a number of special schools of practice based upon different theories of disease. These different schools have now practically disappeared, due partly to the lapse of time, and partly to the unification of opinion with the rapid growth of the sciences underlying medical practice. On the other hand, during the present century there have appeared a number of cults of somewhat similar types, differing from the earlier manifestations in that they rarely assume to be able to deal with all forms of disease. All of them require briefer and much less complete education, and tend, therefore, to be regarded as short cuts to the practice of medicine. The earliest of these was osteopathy, which developed during the latter part of the nineteenth century, and was followed by chiropractic, naturopathy, and others. These groups have sought from the state legislatures licenses, sometimes partial, and sometimes complete, authorizing them to practice medicine or some portion of that field. In various states special boards have been established, while in some others the existing board with additions has to deal with the problem. The chief objection to their existence is that the practice of medicine is thus more or less thrown into the field of politics, and legislative bodies with very incomplete knowledge are asked to pass upon the propriety of giving these groups the security of licensure. It will be noted that such difficulties do not arise under the system of registration, or arise in a minor form. Probably the most serious complication due to the development of these groups, often referred to as cults, is that they have frequently maneuvered the physician into a difficult and undesirable position. The theory of licensure is that it establishes a degree of competence which is minimum for the practice of medicine, and, to that extent, it creates a body with some of the attributes of a monopoly. It is, of course, highly important that the expert opinion of licensed physicians should be at the service of the state in advising as to what are the essential qualifications for modern medical practice and what alterations in the law should from time to time be made in order to keep the practice of medicine abreast of scientific progress. But, on the contrary, it is in no way the duty of physicians to influence the action of legislative bodies except in their capacity as experts. They are under no requirement to protect the public against legislation which may be ill-considered or unwise. Not infrequently it has occurred that the medical profession, acting through its state medical societies, has been maneuvered into a position where it appeared to be more concerned with the exclusion of interlopers than with the fundamental questions of safe medical practice. This has had a tendency to create in the minds of the public a false impression of the position of the medical profession, and to that extent has undermined the security of its position.

The Private Practice of Medicine

In the United States, the practice of medicine in all its fields is, as was above pointed out, under state supervision as provided by licensure. The license to practice is in no way specific and authorizes the physician to practice medicine or surgery either as a whole or in part. Such licensure is based upon the assumption that the graduate, having attained the qualifications specified by the law, may safely be trusted with the general care and oversight of the health of the public. It does not assume, nor tend to assume, any special qualifications above this. Until relatively recent times the overwhelming majority of recent graduates entered general practice, and, until within the last thirty years, practically all specialists developed from general practitioners, who had either found particular interest in a subdivision of the field, or found that it was a sounder economic relation, particularly in the larger centers of population. Within the last twenty years, however, there has developed an increasing number of graduates, who, with either a short period of general practice, or with none at all, undertake postgraduate study for periods of some three to five years, and thus equipped, confine themselves to special fields without previous experience in general practice. There is also a much larger group, who, having as a rule some or considerable experience in general practice, decide to limit their practice, and do so without adequate postgraduate study and without having, in fact, the qualifications which would be recognized either by the profession or by the public as properly antecedent to proclaiming themselves specialists. It is extremely difficult to come to any accurate opinion as to the number of physicians who have limited their practice. Perhaps the best evidence of the tendency in this regard is that shown by recent graduates. Of some interest in this connection is Table I. If this can be taken as a fair cross section of the field, it is very evident that the tendency toward specialization in

TABLE I [*]

SPECIALIZATION AMONG RECENT GRADUATES, BY YEAR OF GRADUATION

TYPE OF PRACTICE	PERCENTAGE DISTRIBUTION		
	1915 GRADUATES	1920 GRADUATES	1925 GRADUATES
ALL TYPES	100.0	100.0	100.0
GENERAL PRACTICE	22.5	23.8	25.1
GENERAL PRACTICE WITH SPECIAL ATTENTION TO SPECIALTY	35.6	40.4	40.5
LIMITED TO SPECIALTY	40.9	35.0	34.0
NOT PRACTICING	1.0	0.8	0.5

whole or in part is very marked, and probably increasing. This table appears to show that less than a quarter of the graduates of fifteen years ago are in general practice, while three-quarters have limited their work, at least to some extent. The apparent diminution in specialization in graduates of only five years is probably a reflection of their relatively recent graduation, which has not allowed them time in which to come to a decision. Even if we assume that the tendency to specialization is very much less than that suggested by this table, we must still regard it as a very important development, and one which must be taken into account in any estimate of the service which physicians of the United States are now offering.

Table II shows the considerable variation of this tendency in different medical schools. Thus, while 36 per cent of recent medical graduates have specialized, those from some of the universities—notably, Johns Hopkins and Harvard—show a relatively very high percentage of specialists. Some other schools—notably, Long Island College of Medicine, University and Bellevue Hospital Medical College, Jefferson Medical College of Philadelphia, and Tufts College Medical School—show a small percentage.

The general practitioner is the natural descendant of the family physician of an earlier age, but, owing to changes in social and economic status, he has a less close contact with his patients than did his predecessor. The behavior of the medical practitioner is chiefly governed by custom and his professional code of ethics, since the law steps in relatively seldom to interfere. Thus, the law assumes that a

TABLE II [5]

SPECIALIZATION AMONG RECENT GRADUATES, BY SCHOOLS

	PER CENT
ALL MEDICAL COLLEGES	36.1
ALBANY MEDICAL COLLEGE	41.8
UNIVERSITY OF BUFFALO SCHOOL OF MEDICINE	26.2
COLUMBIA UNIVERSITY COLLEGE OF PHYSICIANS AND SURGEONS	39.1
HAHNEMANN MEDICAL COLLEGE OF PHILADELPHIA	14.7
HARVARD UNIVERSITY MEDICAL SCHOOL	64.1
HOWARD UNIVERSITY COLLEGE OF MEDICINE	4.6
UNIVERSITY OF ILLINOIS COLLEGE OF MEDICINE	31.1
STATE UNIVERSITY OF IOWA COLLEGE OF MEDICINE	48.9
JEFFERSON MEDICAL COLLEGE OF PHILADELPHIA	26.0
JOHNS HOPKINS UNIVERSITY SCHOOL OF MEDICINE	75.1
LONG ISLAND COLLEGE OF MEDICINE	17.8
UNIVERSITY OF MICHIGAN MEDICAL SCHOOL	43.5
UNIVERSITY AND BELLEVUE HOSPITAL MEDICAL COLLEGE	25.3
UNIVERSITY OF PENNSYLVANIA SCHOOL OF MEDICINE	39.4
UNIVERSITY OF CHICAGO, RUSH MEDICAL COLLEGE	44.5
STANFORD UNIVERSITY SCHOOL OF MEDICINE	55.8
UNIVERSITY OF TORONTO FACULTY OF MEDICINE	36.0
TUFTS COLLEGE MEDICAL SCHOOL	27.5
TULANE UNIVERSITY SCHOOL OF MEDICINE	36.1
UNIVERSITY OF VIRGINIA DEPARTMENT OF MEDICINE	61.5

physician holding himself out as a general practitioner of medicine and surgery will exhibit that degree of skill and knowledge which is the average for physicians working in similar communities. If he does not hold himself out as a specialist, he is not assumed to have the qualifications of a specialist, nor to be required to exhibit them. At an earlier day, and probably up to the present time, in those parts of the country chiefly governed by the old English common law, the courts have repeatedly held that a physician, who declares himself to be a practitioner of medicine and advertises the fact by a sign, cannot refuse to visit a patient when called, unless he is physically incapable of doing so. This but supports generally accepted opinion to the effect that if a physician wishes to practice, he must do so. A considerable amount of misapprehension of the relation of physicians to the public has arisen from the fact that they belong to what, rather vaguely, is known as a profession, and have set up for their guidance a code of ethics. Reduced to its essence, a profession may be defined as a field of human activity in which the chief purpose is the service of the community, with financial gain as a necessarily subordinate consideration. Codes of ethics have characterized most, or all, professional groups and attempt to lay down laws of conduct which shall in general be followed. They have as their chief object the separation of a professional group from a business or trade group, though in recent times there has been a clear tendency in business groups to develop codes of ethics and thus to approach professional standards. Without going into detail, the code of ethics specifies that a physician shall not indulge in advertising, shall respect the rights of other physicians in their patients, and, in general, shall avoid actions which tend to call particular attention to himself or his abilities. Reduced to its simplest terms, it is little more than the codification of the requirements to conduct himself like a gentleman. The chief peculiarity of private practice, as distinguished from other forms of practice later to be discussed, is that the physician in private acts as an individual and is responsible only to the law and the medical customs of the day. It should be borne in mind that repeated court decisions over a long period of years have held that the relation between patient and physician is not a contract, and that the physician does not agree or guarantee to cure, or even to alleviate, but only to treat the patient to the best of his knowledge and ability. If he be in general practice, he is in free and open competition with all other general practitioners and with any or all specialists to the extent that he regards himself as capable of working in their fields. This gives tremendous freedom of action and by the same token throws upon the individual a tremendous, and at times appalling, responsibility for the proper ordering of his conduct.

General Practice

It is not necessary further to define the meaning of the above term, as that point has already been discussed. It will, however, at once be noted that, since the field is general, the position of the general practitioner has undergone marked change during the period of rapid development of scientific knowledge. While thirty years ago it was possible for a single individual to be relatively well informed in the whole field of medical knowledge, such a thing has today become quite unthinkable. Even if at graduation he were thoroughly abreast of current knowledge, which is obviously not the case, a few years in busy practice often leaves him considerably in the rear in many fields, and hopelessly in the rear in some important particulars. Also, at the present time he obviously cannot live unto himself alone, if he is to offer to his patients a reasonable article of service. He has become profoundly dependent upon the factual information which can be obtained from laboratory procedures, many of which he cannot carry out himself. He has come to require relatively close contact with colleagues having special knowledge in various fields, and his use of consultants must be enormously greater than at any previous period. He must not only have access to laboratories and consultants, but to hospitals. If his practice is to remain reasonably abreast of current knowledge, all of these accessories must not only be available, but he must in fact avail himself of them. This requires not only a broad-minded attitude on the part of the physician, but also a public opinion educated to the necessity of providing such adjuncts as laboratories and hospitals, which the physician himself would find quite beyond his means. His task is not made easier by the fact that, since he holds himself out as a general practitioner, his patients have no methods of deciding as to the limits of his capacity. While it is probably true that the average layman assumes himself to be able to select his physician, there is no field in which human judgment is so fallible, and in which it has so little to guide it. It is interesting at this point to note the opinion of a layman, Walton H. Hamilton, who has made some study of the problem.

Although "the personal choice of a physician" is an excellent ideal, it does not, under current conditions, work well in practice. An old maxim, long known to every student of social philosophy, calls for a restriction of personal choice when "the consumer is not a proper judge of the quality of the ware." The art of medicine is intricate; the relation of the treatment of the sick to results obtained cannot be appraised by a layman; in medicine, almost more certainly than anywhere else, the patient has not the knowledge requisite for judgment. In almost every city reputable physicians will admit—at least in private—that the competence of their fellows is not in accord with their respective reputations. Values are treasured long after they have begun to depreciate; and the idea of "free choice" is much too individualistic to be easily surrendered. But its worth is to a large extent fictitious; and the expense and suffering which attends wrong choice and "shopping around" add greatly to the avoidable human costs of medicine.[6]

We have proceeded upon the theory, that each of us can select his physician, largely because at an earlier day medical knowledge was much more incomplete, the education of most physicians was more nearly equal, and, in the long run, the question of personality and strength of character was the largest single consideration. If this ever was a sound basis for judgment, it has long since ceased to be so, and today the public, in its selection of physicians, has so little basis for guidance that, on the whole, there is no presumption that such selection will be made as the result of any intellectual process.

There are other not inconsiderable difficulties which surround the general practice of medicine. If the physician is to practice successfully, as the word is generally and loosely used, he must at least hope to have a large number of patients, but, interestingly enough, the more patients he has, the less possible will it be for him to devote to each one the precise amount of time and care which he might well judge to be desirable. When he does acquire a large practice, his hours are long, he is constantly at the beck and call of everyone who desires his services, and it becomes progressively more difficult for him to devote a reasonable amount of time, if any time at all, to attempting to keep abreast of the rapid changes in medical knowledge. Thus develops the paradox that the busier the practitioner becomes, the more likely he is to fall behind in his knowledge of modern medicine. Of late years, much has been said about the importance of retaining the attributes and the individuality of the so-called family practitioner. To this impossibility, allusion has already been made, but it is continually assumed that the general practitioner by his contact with his patients will acquire a considerably greater insight into their hidden peculiarities than is possible for a specialist or a consultant. This is, of course, a consummation devoutly to be desired, but it is—I believe—less true today in practice than we should like to believe. Just as the turmoil and pressure of general practice make it difficult, or impossible, for the general practitioner to keep track of the game, so it is unwise to assume that his knowledge of the backgrounds and foregrounds of his patients will approach the accuracy which his predecessor, the family physician, commonly achieved.

Another serious problem which he constantly has to face is that of the importance, or desirability, of calling specialists in consultation. If the problem of consultation were only that of requesting assistance when it would be desirable in the interests of his patient, and would reinforce or aid his own judgment, then it would be a comparatively simple one, but it is much more complex. In one way or another, the question of finance has an uncomfortable way of intruding itself. He may be well aware that the economic circumstances of his patient will make the calling of a consultant a considerable burden, and he is torn between the desirability of a consultant and the importance of not dragging his patient toward the poorhouse. There is also another side to the financial difficulty. It is always a fair assumption that the patient, unless in affluent circumstances, has only a limited amount of money which he can afford to spend upon any particular illness. Now the fact is bound to intrude itself into the consciousness of the general practitioner that almost exactly to the extent that he asks for the assistance of a consultant, to that extent will his own fees be diminished. This is but one of the many instances in which the competitive practice of medicine throws a tremendous, and not always well-supported, strain upon the moral fiber of the physician. If he proceeds upon the assumption that his own skill and judgment are sufficient to deal with the problem, he may fall into grave error, to the detriment of his patient, whereas if he make it a general practice to ask for the assistance of consultants whenever he believes it will be to the advantage of his patient, he may easily find himself faced with figurative or actual starvation. This ever-present dilemma is probably accountable, in part, for the tendency of men who have had considerable experience in private practice to contract their field gradually and to become partial or complete specialists, even though their training in the field of specialization has been inadequate. It is largely responsible also for wholly reprehensible practices which have developed, chiefly within the last fifteen or twenty years, and which are known to the public, if at all, under the rather blanket term of "fee-splitting." This point will be discussed later.

It would be improper to conclude even a brief discussion of the position of the general practitioner without pointing out that it is true here, as in most fields, that generalization is notoriously dangerous. Thus, the position actually occupied by the general practitioner may be eminently satisfactory, and he may be able to deliver to his public an article of service which is really good. On the other hand, it may be true that his position is eminently unsatisfactory, that for an enormous variety of reasons, over many of which he has little control, he may find himself in an unsatisfactory position morally, spiritually, and financially, and he may be actually, or vaguely, aware of the fact that he is not able to deliver to his patients the article of service which they need, and which he would like to give them.

The character of his work will vary very much according to his location. In the very large cities many men begin practice as general practitioners and by narrowing their practice to some or a great extent become what in the jargon of the trade is referred to as an internist—though why this utterly obscure phrase has grown up to define the position of one who holds himself out as particularly qualified in the diagnosis of disease, God only knows. In the large cities the percentage of whole or complete specialists has tended to rise rapidly. A recent survey of the situation in Detroit and Philadelphia by Sinai appears to show that in Detroit 58 per cent of the practitioners are more or less specialized, while in Philadelphia the percentage runs to 65.[7] Under conditions in the large cities, the general practitioner will find it increasingly difficult to maintain toward his patients the proper relation of a general adviser, and will of necessity have to deal more largely with an itinerant or floating population. Consequently, his patients come to him more or less by accident. This is obviously an unsatisfactory type of practice both from the point of view of the patient and the physician.

Practice in the smaller cities, from 50,000 to 150,000, is undoubtedly more satisfactory. Here there are enough specialists, but hopefully from his viewpoint not too many. The general practitioner stands a better chance of being able to have a clientele consisting of people whom he sees over a period of years. However, with the occasional rapid changes of population, such as are today not uncommon, he may find himself at any moment in the less desirable position of a general practitioner in a big city.

His position is probably increasingly improved in the smaller cities, which may be defined as those with a population of 20,000 to 50,000. Here his relationship will generally be sounder, and his greatest difficulty may be in finding always at his disposal specialists who are in fact, not in name, qualified to help him out.

We come finally to the position of the general practitioner in the small town. This, in the old days, was the place of development of the family physician. The population was relatively immobile, he knew everybody either by contact or reputation, he frequently, or generally, had important knowledge of their heredity and economic background, and he was in the best possible position to be of service. As already pointed out, the possibility that the general practitioner will today occupy the position which certainly was occupied by his grandfather has become increasingly smaller. The population is somewhat more mobile, in general terms, and, in terms of paved roads and automobiles, is violently more mobile. At the earlier day he could generally supply those things necessarily prerequisite to medical diagnosis and treatment. Today he obviously cannot do so, and must have the assistance of laboratories and consultants, which may be hard to obtain. Finally, his assurance of making a living is considerably less than it used to be, and, as a consequence, the probability of being able to keep a wife about the house approaches the vanishing point. It thus appears that when we talk about the position of the general practitioner in the field of medicine, we really are not talking about anything in particular. If we desire to come to accurate conclusions as to the position which he now occupies, and the position which we desire that he should occupy, if complete and satisfactory medical service is to be had at all economic levels, then, obviously, we must define our terms—or we shall fall into the traps which have so commonly ensnared those who attempt to solve complicated problems with glittering generalities.

INCOME OF GENERAL PRACTITIONERS

Since, by definition, the general practitioner is the person whom it would be desirable to have in relation to the patient at the earliest moment and most continuously, and since it is true that he cannot, by definition, supply all of the special skill and knowledge which may be desirable, it is fairly clear that he must depend for his support upon fees relatively small as compared with the specialist, and, hence, that he must have a good many of them. As a necessary and probable consequence of this situation there arises the conflict, already referred to, under which he is constantly at the beck and call of everybody who desires his services. He is under tremendous pressure to see a large number of people. This carries with it the risk, difficult to avoid, of exercising a considerable amount of guesswork, which, however deified, leaves him in a position not far removed from that of his predecessor, who dealt largely in guesswork because, forsooth, he had nothing better to offer. Today the scientific basis of medicine has been pushed to a point where guesswork is rarely necessary, yet, the temptation to indulge in it may readily strain human resistance.

V

SPECIALISTS AND GROUP MEDICINE

Special practice, or specialization, is nothing but a translation into action of the inevitable forces making for subdivision of labor, which have been operating, progressively and increasingly, since the Industrial Revolution. Of course, specialization did not begin at any particular time, and we are well aware that even in the Middle Ages there were practitioners of what might, by a stretch of the imagination, be called medicine whose whole offering consisted in a willingness to "cut for stone." One need not press the point that subdivision of labor, another phrase for specialization, has sprung from a rapid increase of scientific knowledge, and it is in no way peculiar to the practice of medicine. In fact, it is probably true that there are more narrow specialists outside of the field of medicine than in it.

Special Practice

Thirty years ago specialization in medicine had not gone far. In general, there were the general medical consultants, the general surgical consultants or general surgeons, and the specialists in diseases of the eye, ear, nose, and throat. Steadily, however, the growing amount of scientific knowledge and the importance of developing special fields led to increasing subdivision, which has now gone to a great length. In the field of medicine there still remains what is commonly referred to as the internist. He is practically the counterpart of the general medical consultant, and is a type of general practitioner who, however, is chiefly concerned with studying difficult problems and acting as what might be called senior counsel in the case. At times, the internist acts chiefly as a very high grade diagnostician to whom patients come, or are referred, in difficult cases, and upon whom often rests the responsibility of advising consultation with various specialists. The fact that he acts importantly as a consultant operates to reduce the number of patients that he must see, and thereby enables him to give to each more thorough and complete study. He is also, by definition, closely in touch with the laboratory and with capable special advisers. One is tempted to think of him as the modern development of the general practitioner and to entertain the, perhaps futile, hope that the time may not be too distant when the general practitioner will occupy this position and be able to devote to each patient an amount of time backed by special advice, which will more certainly lead to accurate opinions. The subdivisions of the field of medicine are numerous and increasing. Among the best known is the splitting off of diseases of children from general medical practice, a form of specialization which has certainly operated immensely to the benefit of the rising generation and has much diminished infant mortality. Diseases of the skin have also become a subdivision of medicine, with which, in the past, the management of syphilis has commonly been combined. More and more, however, syphilis is being regarded as a special field, to the extent that it cannot be satisfactorily managed by the general practitioner. Special groups also concern themselves with diseases of the heart, with diseases of the lungs—and here the increase in our ability to manage pulmonary tuberculosis has been very importantly fostered by the work of specialists. A group has also developed for the care of diseases of the gastro-intestinal tract.

It is, however, in the field of surgery that the greatest number of special divisions have developed—though a great deal of the work does not specifically concern itself with surgical operations. Thus, there are a good many surgeons, particularly in the large cities, who confine themselves almost exclusively to abdominal surgery. Obstetrics and gynecology, either separate or combined, constitute a well-developed group. Orthopedic surgery has achieved an established position, and is tending to take over certain portions of the field of the general surgeon, particularly in the management of difficult fractures. The surgery of the genito-urinary tract, more recently referred to as urology, is a well-established specialty, and the specialties dealing with the organs of special sense, the eye and the ear, together with the nose and the throat, have continued to separate themselves more and more from general medicine and general surgery. During the last twenty years, there has developed a small though very important specialty dealing with diseases of the brain and nervous system, which has resulted in enormous advances in this field. Even further subdivisions might be noted, but these are perhaps sufficient to indicate that in surgery, where niceties of technic and prolonged technical experience are at a premium, specialization has, on the whole, gone further than in the field of general medicine. The general surgeon still exists, though there are an increasing number of fields in which he finds it difficult to keep abreast of the times.

Allusion has already been made to the general causes of the development of specialization, and the distinction between the well-qualified and ill-qualified specialists has been pointed out. It is perhaps wise, at this time, to discuss briefly what may properly be held as the necessary training for qualified specialists in many of these fields. Certainly, specialization should not be undertaken without a broad basic hospital experience, and a good case can be made for the view that a period of experience in the general practice of medicine of something like two years is much to be desired. However, special training, which will qualify these physicians as experts upon whom the public may rely, will require at least three years of intensive study under excellent conditions. These conditions will require hospital affiliations, and what amounts practically to apprenticeship to finished experts. In the group loosely referred to as the medical specialties, three years is perhaps sufficient, but it may fairly be doubted whether this is a sufficient length of time to really qualify men in the surgical specialties, particularly those requiring an unusual knowledge and dexterity. For example, a training in the field of general surgery can probably be satisfactorily obtained in five years, including the preliminary hospital experience, but excluding any time devoted to general practice outside of the hospital.

The specialist in the fields of the special senses will probably require more time. The urologist should, I believe, be a fairly capable general surgeon before he undertakes the often complicated and trying surgical problems of the genito-urinary system. In the same way, the orthopedist should be a surgeon before he is a specialist, and five years will probably be less than will commonly be thought necessary for his development. In the narrower fields, as typified by the surgery of the nervous system, prolonged experience is necessary because the opportunities for broad experience will be more difficult to obtain, and a really comprehensive view, therefore, will take more time.

It is clear that a training of this kind will be a considerable economic burden, but it may be quite dogmatically asserted that the public is entitled to be assured that those who hold themselves out as experts in special fields shall have very much more to offer than a broad general training. Some interesting educational problems present themselves in connection with the requirement that specialists should really know their business. The educational facilities of the country are today doubtfully able to offer the training which they ought to have to the number of people who will be really needed in these special fields. There is clear evidence, however, that this weakness in postgraduate education is being slowly but surely remedied, and it is probably true that today the hospitals and organized postgraduate schools of the country could come very near to supplying the necessary number of qualified specialists.

INCOME OF SPECIALISTS

It seems tolerably obvious that the remuneration of the properly qualified specialist should be relatively large, not only on account of the unavoidable expense of his education, but because it is likely that he will then be able to see, in a satisfactory manner, a number of patients relatively small as compared with the general practitioner. If one were able to allocate the remuneration of the general practitioner and the specialist through the medium of an unprejudiced body, there would probably be relatively little disagreement, but that, of course, would be purely utopian. The fact remains that the fees of the specialist are relatively large—often out of proportion to those of general practitioners, particularly in view of the fact that as far as the public is concerned there is no means of distinguishing between the fully qualified and the poorly qualified expert. From this inevitable, and at times commercial, disagreement between the general practitioner and the specialist—and because of the conviction of the public that they are entitled to consult specialists with or without previous competent medical advice—there has arisen a most difficult and, at times, unsavory state of affairs in regard to professional charges, which will require separate discussion.

Group Practice [1]

The tendency of physicians to group themselves together in such a way as to offer a more complete and varied service to patients is a relatively modern development. Though, superficially, it might be regarded as the outgrowth of associations properly spoken of as partnerships, this is, I think, not the case. Partnerships of more or less loose types have existed in medical practice for many years, following the example of other professional groups, notably the law. However, these partnerships, as a rule, concern themselves chiefly, or entirely, with the increase of the amount of service which can be rendered, rather than in offering varieties of service which is characteristic of the group. Thus, a busy practitioner might associate with himself one or more younger men under partnership agreements, but, thereby, he only extended the type of practice which he was carrying on and did not add importantly to its variety. In the same way, it has been the custom of surgeons, both in the general and special field, to associate with themselves younger men, sometimes under partnership agreements. This was done only for the purpose of enabling them more effectively to carry on the same type of work which they had been doing alone. There is, I believe, a clear distinction between what is properly spoken of as group practice and the earlier, and still continuing, system of partnerships.

Obviously, groups are, or may be, of many kinds, and it is important to define the types of grouping with which we are concerned. Group practice, in general, might be held to cover such associations of practitioners as are found in the government services where a group of physicians on a salary basis is concerned with the care of large numbers of people. In a sense, the physicians and surgeons practicing in large charity hospitals constitute a group in that they spread the benefit of their various experiences among each other to the advantage of the patient. But, though these developments have some of the characteristics of group practice, they are not those with which we are chiefly concerned. The outstanding importance of the grouping together of physicians representing different fields of medicine has been its value as an experiment in widening the sphere of the individual, but still retaining the essential characteristics of private practice.

This development has evidently come about as the result of changing conditions of two kinds—medical and economic. The medical reason for the development of the group is the self-evident fact that the individual practitioner is in constant need of advice and assistance from colleagues who have devoted their time to special fields. The conception thus arose that the effectiveness of the general practitioner might be increased by directly associating with himself the commonly necessary special consultants. Assuming good judgment in the selection of the group, no argument is necessary to show that it can offer a superior grade of service.

On the economic side, a wisely arranged association of general and special practitioners will obviously have the result of making possible very large savings in overhead, which, today, particularly in the case of the specialist, has become a very important charge against his gross income. That this does, in fact, occur has been frequently denied, chiefly by the various groups commonly referred to as "organized medicine." Quite recently the first Minority Report of the Committee on the Costs of Medical Care made a flat denial of this assertion. Recent careful study of at least three large private groups shows that they are able to offer high grade service at less cost than that being offered in several large cities. That the formation of a group does in some magical way alter the individual characteristics of its members is not here asserted, but it is asserted that by sound organization the group can much diminish overhead charges. Insofar as decrease in expense for overhead operates to increase the net income of the group, it will be possible for the group to offer their services to the community at a lower figure. This amounts, of course, simply to passing on to the consumer the benefits obtained by better organization, a maxim which has dominated business for many years.

Many, or perhaps most, of the groups which have thus grown up have taken the form of corporate entities, but such an arrangement is by no means necessary, and has not been universally employed. It is, perhaps, the narrowest and most concrete form of group practice, but one might easily enlarge the concept by adding to it the very loose association of practitioners about a community hospital. There is evidently an increasing tendency of physicians to group themselves about hospitals, to the extent of having their offices in the immediate neighborhood, or even in the hospital itself. This is evidence of their desire to avail themselves of the technical equipment of the hospital in various laboratory services. Such a physical association has often led to a loose type of professional association under which consultation was much more readily available, and the proper adjustment of professional charges easier. One may easily look forward to an increase of this tendency toward loose, voluntary, and probably changeable, association as carrying with it a good many of the advantages which accrue from the more formal corporate groups.

The tendency toward grouping, formal and informal, is also important as showing evidence of the appreciation within the profession itself of the physical difficulties of translating the outward forms of the medical practice of an earlier day into the complicated environment of modern medicine. If skillfully employed, it can easily have the result of retaining all of the important elements of individual thought and action, and enabling the members constantly to check their own opinions by those of their more expert colleagues, and, perhaps even more important, enabling the whole group to keep themselves more nearly in step with modern progress, by association of specialist and "generalist."

As has already been intimated, the principal development, particularly of the formal groups, has occurred since 1918. The earliest, and most outstanding, of these groups is the Mayo Clinic, beginning in 1887, and from this has probably come the tendency of group practice to develop most rapidly and most extensively in the Northwest and the Middle West. Undoubtedly, the subdivision of the medical work incident to service during the War also tended to suggest to practitioners, who in civil life had been working independently, that they could improve their work by some type of combination. There are, at the present time, about 150 such groups, covering a very wide area, and exhibiting considerable variation in type of organization. In general, however, they undertake to carry on the general practice of medicine, although a fair number of them at least include dentistry in their offering. Also the staffs are generally on a salary basis, but divided into owners and non-owners. This, of course, reflects their origin, in that, as a rule, one or more individual practitioners undertook to start the group, often invested a considerable amount of their own capital, and, therefore, have retained a controlling interest in the business. Almost universally, they have employed lay business managers who have charge of the regulation of fees, the buying of equipment, and the general commercial aspects of the establishment. Many of the groups employ several business men in their establishments. They universally employ some non-medical personnel to carry on the laboratory and allied functions. Since they undertake to offer general medical care, their organization is generally based upon providing more physicians skilled in general practice than in the special fields. Their plans, as a rule, provide that the patient shall be seen in the first instance by the general physician, who then calls for such special advice as seems to him required. In this way, the pattern which has proved sound in medical practice is to a considerable extent retained. In the smaller groups it is not always possible to provide specialists in all of the commoner fields, and, to this extent, they may be unable to offer the most complete type of service. They do, however, almost always have a sufficient number of specialists so that the opinions given by the group will represent a very satisfactory offering in medical service.

One of the questions most commonly raised in regard to the ultimate value and success of this type of practice concerns itself with the extent to which the personal relation between patient and physician will be lost. Thus, it has been asserted that this type of practice necessarily involved the loss of personal relation, and, to that extent, undermined the whole basis of private practice. A survey of the opinions of physicians engaged in this type of work shows that they do not believe this necessarily results. My own experience has convinced me that the extent to which the relation is lost, or maintained, will depend almost entirely upon the personnel of the group, and very little upon the type of organization. I believe it quite beyond question that if the group really desires to maintain a high grade of personal relation, similar to that which exists in average private practice, it can do so without difficulty. In this connection, it is well to remember that in a great deal of medical practice today the personal relation has dropped into the background. Many patients consult physicians without any intention of consulting them again. The patient of today is inclined to select different physicians for different types of service, and is less impressed than in the past with the view that a general practitioner can wisely guide him through the intricacies of the modern management of disease.

There is another aspect of the group type of practice which may become increasingly important in the future. A good many of these groups have entered into various contractual relations with organizations in the community. This is based upon a definite contract by which the group undertakes to offer various types of service, from merely ambulatory or office treatment up to complete medical oversight, care, and hospitalization, the charges varying with the type of service offered. This is an attempt to utilize the group as a basis for the development of medical care on a prepayment basis. Without taking up at this time a discussion which will later have to be developed further, it seems proper to suggest that the offering of medical service on a contract basis by private groups has outstanding advantages over its offering by business organizations, in which expenses not medical in character are bound to be incurred. Though it might be expected that the medical profession, as a whole, would recognize the advantage of this type of contract offered by their own members instead of by business organizations, "organized medicine" has not looked with favor, up to the present time, on such contractual relations and has seriously interfered with their development.

The time which has elapsed since any considerable number of these private group organizations have been in operation is too short to warrant an entirely sound estimate of the place which they will occupy in the future. Nevertheless, they certainly offer an interesting bit of experimental work along a line where factual information is very important. The survey undertaken under the auspices of the Committee on the Costs of Medical Care has brought the facts well up to date, but they are too meager to warrant any dogmatic assertions. Though, as has been frequently pointed out by their critics, many groups have been unable to withstand the recent economic and financial storms, this should not be held as evidence of their economic impermanence. Few of them had lived through previous economic convulsions, and their organizations were not planned with this in view. It is, I believe, as unsound to point to their failure to weather this storm as it would be to point to the failure of thousands of banks, as evidence that banks were an unsound economic development. A dispassionate review of the evidence which has been accumulating during the last fifteen years appears to me to show conclusively that the principle involved in group practice is fundamentally sound and that the groups are certain to increase in number. So wise an observer as Sir Arthur Newsholme, who can hardly be accused of overrating this development, which has but just started in Great Britain, has this to say on the general principle:

It may be accepted, then, as axiomatic that *adequate medical care for a large proportion of the total number of sick persons necessitates the organization of measures and of institutions beyond the power of the individual private medical practitioner to provide.* [And again]: When local medical practitioners have learned the fundamental lesson that, in modern circumstances, *if the family is to continue to be the unit of medical practice, then a team of medical practitioners, and not an isolated practitioner, should be the unit on the medical side,* this and allied coöperative work will become practicable, at least in populous districts.[2]

Personally, I should prefer to go further and say that, under modern conditions, first-class medical care not only to the family but to the individual requires a team, and not an isolated practitioner.

I cannot follow the conclusion expressed in the *Minority Report* of the Committee on the Costs of Medical Care when it refers to private group clinics:

That it has accomplished generally or can ever accomplish what is there claimed for it is open to grave doubt. There is nothing in our own experience nor have we been able to find anything in the Committee's studies to lead us to conclude that group practice can furnish in general better or cheaper medical care than we have at present.[3]

Rexwald Brown, speaking with some knowledge of group practice, disagrees with this view. He says:

Group medical practice is predicated on the belief that professional duties are paramount to professional rights. . . .

Intelligent group practice comprehends organization methods and ability but not of the old type which breeds uniformity of thought and action. Well-managed group guidance tries to keep alive the creative spirit of originality in the organization. . . .

Soundly thinking medical groups are not concerned over professional rights as much as the members of a county medical society are. Groups have more time to grasp an understanding of what lay people are striving for and are more likely to have social sympathies. In groups the personal profit attitude of mind is replaced by the growth of a policy of adequate compensation, which means satisfactory living conditions to each member of the group. The adequate pay system increases in amount from year to year incident to the development of confidence on the part of the public in the group endeavors.

Group medical practice feels it is better able to make modern medical knowledge applicable to all people than is the individual doctor. If all the doctors of a group think they can, and are desirous of doing so, they can make available to the rich, the poor, and the indigent the priceless treasures of scientific medicine.

In medical groups a new point of view can easily arise in regard to medical ethics. Medical society members usually look upon medical ethics as a crystallization of their rights. Many of the laity look upon medical ethics as often inimical to their rights as human beings. They think of doctors as claimants of a superior class invested with special privileges. These divergent opinions are certainly a clash. The facts are that the medical code largely regulates the professional contacts of doctors with each other. Medical ethics is more concerned with professional etiquette than it is with fundamental morality. Herein is the conflict over medical ethics between doctors and the lay public. Doctors in medical groups, divorced of the onerous burden of providing homes, food, and clothing for the family will be more patient of the feelings of the public.

Group medical practice is evidence of the worth of consultation among doctors. Consultation has been used by individual doctors and exacted by sick patients for centuries. Group practice is an expanded consultation plan. . . .

A new idea is becoming current. Signs of the times are that there is gradual dislodgment of the validity of the teaching that confidence in the chosen doctor may be relied on. Reputable physicians know that the competence of many of their fellows does not measure up to their reputations. The intelligent public is realizing that it is not a proper judge of the qualifications of doctors in respect to judgment, professional morals, modern knowledge of medicine and medical and surgical skill. Freedom of choice of physicians and confidence in the object of choice may easily be delusions. There is a marked difference between confidence in the doctor established on gracious manners and charm of personality and established on diagnostic ability and knowledge of how to apply the armamentaria of treatment. . . .

The present medical unit of action of operation, the County Medical Society, will be broken up into smaller units. This dissolution will occur because a county medical unit is frequently a static body imposing taboos and punishment on all suggestions of an experimental nature. The smaller units will be medical groups organized on lines of furthering creative thought in its membership. . . .

Group practices will demonstrate that graduation from a medical school, license to practice medicine granted by the State and membership in a county medical society are not satisfactory criteria of the competency and responsibility of the doctor. Group membership will mean the measuring up to contributions of worth in the development of the group and of society. Among these contributions of worth are repeated examinations for physicians after graduation to determine their knowledge of the steady advancement in medical circles. A control of this character would be assurance to a patient that a doctor of his choice is a good choice. . . .

Group physicians are taught to have a larger understanding of the meaning of scientific medicine. . . . Their idea of medical services is not bound up with business methods.

This conception of service rather than personal profit is solidifying the pathway of group practice. The setup of group practice, fashioned around the general practitioner, nowadays called the internist, is the answer to the perplexing question agitating the general practitioner and the specialist. . . . The specialists are the hands of the internists. This method of integration between general practitioner, the trusted guide, counselor and friend of the patient and the specialist, who applies modern medical knowledge and skill in a superior way to the interests of the patient, is the type of collaboration this new era, looking into the future, needs.[4]

It appears to me to be of the first importance that we should consider very carefully the ultimate possibilities of group practice, particularly if we look forward to the development in this country of some plan which is suited to our own state of social progress, and is based upon developments which have already taken place here. It should not be forgotten that the development of the group is not only peculiar to this country, but is the single outstanding contribution of the medical profession to improved organization for the delivery of medical service.

There are certain underlying principles which will be required for the development of successful groups. They must be composed of like-minded people who are profoundly impressed with the ideals of service, and are seeking an opportunity to so organize their work that they may be relieved, as far as possible, from the strains and stresses of commercial competition. The members of a group should have, I think, a broader grasp of the problems of economics than is the rule among physicians. A group is not a satisfactory medium for the development of the highly individual practitioner, or one with the attributes of the prima donna. Such people, though of enormous value in any profession, must in the long run live alone. The personnel of a successful group must be willing to subordinate their individual preferences to an extent greater than is always seen among professional people. This subordination must be concerned, however, only with the problems of normal adjustment, and need not—in fact should not—involve questions of principle.

There are certain requirements on the economic side which will be necessary in the future development of group practice. The evidence is quite sufficient to show that, by this type of organization, unit costs in the delivery of high-grade medical service can be importantly reduced. At the present time, charges, if not costs, for really first-class medical service have risen to a point where they are being affected by the law of diminishing returns. It is quite certain that further attention to the cutting of unit costs will enable groups to offer service at a lower rate, and thereby widen their sphere of usefulness. Study of the difficulties of at least several groups appears to me to show that they have failed to grasp this and other well-known economic laws. They have often failed to appreciate the importance of adequate reserves. They have tended to spend their money as do individual practitioners—as they get it, without sufficient thought for the morrow. For this reason, it will be important to include in the organization of groups a handsome proportion of long-headed laymen—people not only competent to handle the details of business organization, but also competent to keep the group in close touch with prevailing public opinion. Organized on these principles they can maintain the ideals of personal service, and yet keep step with the economic changes of the day to an extent which has not been characteristic of the practice of medicine by individuals.

The objections to group practice such as those voiced by the first *Minority Report,* referred to above, are not, I think, based upon evidence of medical or economic failure, but really upon evidence of success and fear of change. What the *Minority Report* seeks is to perpetuate an organization of individuals, which seems to me to run grave danger of developing along the line of a trade union. In fact, this has taken place in France, through the development of medical syndicalism. It might even develop toward an organization of the old guild type, which was, in fact, an attempt to maintain the position of the individual in disregard of his relation to society. Too violent an attempt to maintain the individual organizations of the past is likely to result in a self-centered use of the ethics of the profession. One sees in certain foreign countries, particularly in France, the struggle of the profession to maintain its organizations of individuals, by using certain of its ethical standards as a cloak for incompetence. Thus, in France, the doctrine of the privileged communication has been used as a support for incompetence and a cloak for shoddy work. On this point I quote from Newsholme:

My own opinion on this discussion can be stated in the words of Professor Barthélemy, a distinguished French jurist, and of Dr. Rist, a distinguished physician in Paris. Professor Barthélemy very properly says medical secrecy paralyses justice ("La règle du secret énerve la justice"); and Dr. Rist states his conviction that "the doctrine of absolute medical secrecy supplies a means of escaping cases of conscience, of declining responsibility, and of washing one's hands of the most obvious duties." This appears to be in his view the true reason for the passionate adhesion of so many doctors to this doctrine.[5]

On the part of organized medicine, too great an insistence on the perpetuation of the present order is in danger of developing into a struggle for the perpetuation of a vested interest.

Of course, the mere fact that medicine has been practiced in a certain pattern for a long period is not an objection to such a plan. I believe it to be the duty of organized medicine to express its opinion clearly and to leave no doubt, in the mind of the public, as to its views of the value of present types of organization. It should be remembered, however, that the decision as to what pattern medical practice will gradually assume will not be made, in the long run, solely upon the opinion of the profession. In this field physicians have no exclusive rights to the expression of authoritative opinion. The problems are economic and social, rather than technical and professional. In the long run, the decision must remain with public opinion, since, after all, it is the public, and not the profession, which is most vitally concerned. I cannot subscribe to the view that any group in the community has any rights which the public is bound to respect, if they can be shown to be opposed to the public interest. The public, to use the economic phrase, is the consumer, and the consumer must in the long run decide the quality and availability of the article in question. There is some evidence that organized medicine is in danger of overlooking this fundamental right of the consumer. We shall be well-advised to distinguish carefully between those fields in which professional opinion is controlling and those in which it carries no weight, except insofar as it does represent average public opinion.

VI

GROUP HEALTH SERVICES

A form of group medical practice which has been developed in this country, and which has provided interesting data on the problem of group management of health is shown by the health services at large universities.

University Health Service

In important particulars, university health service differs from the organization of private group clinics, since it is undertaken by universities which may or may not be tax-supported institutions. The staffs are composed of physicians, some of whom are employed as full-time and some as part-time officers. The greatest value of this development probably lies in the extent to which it contributes evidence of the possibility of supplying high-grade medical supervision and care at a relatively low cost. This has a bearing on the whole problem of group medicine, since it is important to have evidence that group practice can not only deliver a very excellent article of service, but also can do so at low cost, under favorable conditions. It is for this reason that I have included, at this point, a brief survey of university health services. The first large undertaking in this regard was at the University of California, in 1900.[1] They are now being carried on to a considerable extent in many universities. In cases where the medical school is closely associated with the rest of the university, the presence of the teaching staff of the medical school facilitates the maintenance of high-grade medical personnel, which might otherwise be less easy. However, at several universities, very complete arrangements have been made quite apart from the medical school. This gives us an opportunity to see the workings of the plan under both conditions.

A recent survey of the health services at six universities (Cornell, Yale, University of Michigan, University of Minnesota, University of California, and the Oregon Agricultural College) is interesting because in three (Yale, Michigan, and Minnesota) the association with the medical school is more or less intimate, while in the other three (Cornell, California, and Oregon) the organization is entirely separate.[2] These health services undoubtedly began under the stimulus of the necessity of caring for acutely ill students who frequently were without either the means or the information which would procure for them satisfactory medical care. In the process of development, however, they have come very much further, and often undertake a complete preliminary survey of the student on admission. Some of them continue with compulsory periodic check-ups, and all of them offer what might be called dispensary service for the milder types of disease and disability. They have also provided in many instances for room calls, though often a small extra charge is made for these. Many provide hospital care with quite complete specialist service, either within the basic charge or with very moderate addition.

The per capita cost naturally varies within rather wide limits. It is interesting that of the six referred to above, the four state-supported institutions have a per capita cost running very close together, that at California being $16.78, while that at Oregon, $9.66. Of these charges, a large portion is paid by the student, the small balances, varying from $2.10 at California to ten cents at Oregon, being borne by the university. In the case of the two endowed universities a large amount is carried by university funds. Thus, at Yale the high per capita cost of $33.98 is allocated, $20.25 to the student, and $13.73 from university funds, while at Cornell the high rate of $27.59 is allocated, $15.51 to the student, and $12.08 to the university. The apparently high rate at Yale is, at least partly, accounted for by the very extensive investigation which has been made there into the problem of mental hygiene. This is a field in which relatively little has been done by organized groups, and, hence, its cost is disproportionately large. If one studies the amounts paid by the students, one finds that they range from $20.25 at Yale to $9.56 at Oregon. In consideration of the very complete care given, this does not seem excessive.

We may, I think, safely conclude that the health services now undertaken by many universities have very outstanding advantages. Dealing as they do with a group of young people, they are in a position to offer very valuable health education which will undoubtedly be passed on to the general population. They are in a position to make, and do in fact make, thorough periodic examinations. If we are to convince the public of the real value of this type of examination, there is perhaps no better way to do it. Beyond these educational and prophylactic services they also offer care which must certainly be judged to be first-class. Finally, the per capita cost to the individual is not high, and, by its spread over the student body, produces an income sufficient to provide for the maintenance of a satisfactory staff.

It is, of course, true that the conclusions which safely may be drawn from such undertakings are limited. The people with whom they deal are of a narrow age group, and are less likely to show many of the serious disabilities which would develop in other age groups. They cannot, therefore, be taken as evidence that an equally satisfactory grade of care could be offered to a cross-section of the population at a corresponding rate. Nevertheless, in that they, so to speak, catch the patient at an impressionable age and are in a position to develop in him health consciousness and a knowledge, which may easily prove to be of far-reaching importance, of what constitutes satisfactory medical care, they have a value which would accrue in dealing with few other groups.

Industrial Medicine

The term "industrial medicine" is often used to describe two very different things: (1) It may be used to describe a subdivision, or specialty, in medical practice; or (2) it may be used to describe medical service offered in connection with industry.

In the first sense, it concerns itself chiefly with the questions of education, qualifications, and activities of physicians engaged in supervising the medical problems of industry. This branch of medicine, which has now reached the state where it may properly be regarded as constituting a definite specialty, developed largely as a result of the requirements of the Workmen's Compensation Acts. But, even before the passage of these acts, the problems of the industrialist in connection with liability insurance had given rise to increasingly frequent surveys and studies of the medical problems more or less peculiar to industry. However, the passage of workmen's compensation acts by various states created a situation where expert medical service in connection with industry was clearly required if only for economic reasons. At first, these services were concerned chiefly with the immediate care of accident and injury. They, then, developed along the lines of measures to diminish and avoid accident, and, next, into a study by prospective employers of the physical condition of their employees at the time of employment. Under workmen's compensation acts it became of prime importance to avoid the employment of individuals not in reasonably sound physical condition, and certainly not the subject of abnormality which might render the industry liable for compensation. The next development was the inquiry into the existence of occupational disease, more or less inherent in particular industries, and a study of such factory conditions as tended to diminish, or to avoid, those diseases. It will be evident that the field of activity of the physician doing industrial work is very wide.

It is important to note at this time that the impelling reasons for the introduction and development of this branch of medical practice were economic. It could readily be demonstrated that medical supervision might easily result in very large savings, not only in the field of injury and disease for which compensation might be required, but also in the way of reducing the amount of time lost through injuries not requiring compensation. Among the immediate and obvious savings may be listed the value of a careful physical examination, which excluded handicapped people at the time of employment. In this way, the presence of incipient disease, which later might become a charge against industry, also could sometimes be detected. The prompt and satisfactory care of minor industrial accidents was shown to be a very large improvement over previous conditions in which the employee sought out his own medical adviser, and often obtained treatment only after the loss of valuable time. In many industries, conditions of ventilation and hygiene in the plant itself, and inherent in the peculiar industry, were shown to be causes of much lost time, and, thus, of industrial waste. Finally, may be listed the study of specific diseases quite peculiar to industry, the very nature of which were only vaguely understood, until the development of large-scale industry made the causal conditions more evident. These aspects of the problem of industrial medicine were regarded as primarily the concerns of the business itself. Primarily, they were dealt with from the side of management, not from the side of medical care.

Medical Aspects of Industrial Disease

It will be obvious at once that in industry there is an immense variety of medical problems, partly related to injury, and partly to conditions inherent in various occupations. It has not, I think, been sufficiently realized that here has gradually developed a field of medicine which is quite as truly a specialty as many other fields which have long been so recognized.

Dr. Don B. Lowe describes it as follows:

Far and wide, for a long period of time, the industrial physician and surgeon has been supposed to be a combination, civil, mechanical, heating, lighting, ventilating, and chemical engineer; economist, welfare worker, athletic director, public health officer, insurance expert, and sanitary policeman, not to mention a few other conferred titles.[8]

That such a situation requires special training and special experience is obvious, but it is a curious fact that the medical profession has only in very recent times recognized these special problems, and has from the beginning tended to look somewhat askance at the industrial physician or surgeon—apparently because he has left the fold of private practice and open competition, and aligned himself with the forces of industry. One cannot avoid feeling that some of the criticisms which have been leveled by the medical profession at the industrialists have arisen largely because of the detached attitude of the profession itself, and, often, because of its frank hostility to the plans being made by industry in an attempt to improve the condition of its employees.

Various Types of Industrial Medical Service

These vary very widely. In the early days, and to some extent at the present time, the development has gone no further than the part-time employment by a business concern of a general practitioner, often assisted by a trained nurse, and a more or less trained orderly. Under these circumstances, the medical care is largely confined to an incomplete physical examination of candidates for employment, the care of injuries and illness taking place at the plant itself, and a rather incomplete, and sketchy study of hygienic conditions. The better developed organizations will show at least a full-time medical director, with a better-equipped staff and an organization capable of giving satisfactory immediate attention to minor injuries. They may also provide some study of plant conditions, and a fairly complete knowledge of the unusual risks and hazards of the business. Finally, one may note the development of very complete medical establishments, some of which limit their work to immediate care of injury and accident and thorough examination of employees, tending to develop the physical findings, but not undertaking to offer treatment. These more elaborate establishments commonly conduct studies of industrial disease, and have made very important contributions to the knowledge of the subject. The most elaborate organizations include complete medical care for employees and, in some instances, for their family and dependents. This may include office care, home visits, hospital care, and convalescent care.

It is not intended here to go into any extensive study of the present development of industrial medicine, but only to indicate the lines along which progress has been made, to discuss some of the most elaborate offerings of medical service, and, in general, to lay the groundwork for further discussion of the possible place of industrial medicine in a well-rounded offering of medical service at all levels. Three examples of extensive or complete medical service will be briefly noted.

THE ENDICOTT JOHNSON WORKERS MEDICAL SERVICE [4]

The Endicott Johnson Corporation is a large and prosperous corporation situated in Binghamton, Johnson City, Endicott, and Owego, New York. It is engaged in the manufacture of shoes and the tanning of leather. The data which will be given below are those of the company in 1928. At that time, the corporation employed some 15,000 people, had assets valued at $26,000,000.00, and had net sales amounting to more than $69,000,000.00. The medical service began in 1916, probably under the influence of the Workmen's Compensation Act, with a staff of one full-time physician and one nurse. It was, at that time, the intention to care for conditions involving compensation, and to offer medical service to employees who were unable to pay for medical care. Very shortly, the employees requested more service on the ground that they could not afford to pay for care elsewhere. By 1918 the corporation found it difficult to tell who could afford to pay and who could not, and decided to extend the service to all employees desiring it. In 1928 they employed a full-time staff of more than one hundred people. These included twenty-eight physicians, four dentists, five dental hygienists, two physical therapists, sixty-seven trained nurses, four bacteriologists, four pharmacists, seventeen technicians, and sixteen clerks and office assistants. In that year, the medical service included 87,400 house calls and 118,740 office visits. The total cost of the service to the corporation in that year was over $800,000.00. For their hospital care, they made use of three hospitals not owned or controlled by the corporation—one in Binghamton, one in Johnson City, and one in Endicott. They offered complete medical service to the employees and their dependents. The employees were under no compulsion, and might utilize the service or consult their own physicians as they wished. In practice, it appears that nearly 94 per cent of the employees use the service either in whole or in part. Probably over 80 per cent use the service exclusively.

The medical staff.—There were twenty-eight physicians on full-time salary. Of these, fifteen were general practitioners, four were partly specialized, and nine were specialists. It is the custom of the service to encourage outside consultations with other physicians in these localities. In some fields much of the work is done by physicians not directly employed by the company. Thus, most of the urology and most of the orthopedic surgery was handled by outside physicians. In case of emergencies, or when the staff of the service was otherwise employed, private physicians are frequently called, and the relations appear to be cordial.

Salaries.—The salaries of the full-time medical staff vary from $3,000.00 to $12,900.00. Twenty-one, or over 80 per cent, received between $3,000.00 and $7,000.00. One, or 3.8 per cent, received between $9,000.00 and $11,000.00, and four, or over 15 per cent, received between $11,000.00 and $13,000.00, These are net, not gross, incomes, and therefore will compare favorably with the average earnings of physicians doing similar work.

This staff is well-trained and competent, as judged by modern standards of medical education and capacity. Their relation to the individual employees is a personal one, and it is the rule that, if an employee prefers one member of the staff to another, he shall be allowed to employ him within the limits of that physician's working capacity. It is also the rule that an employee shall remain under the care of the same physician. As already pointed out, consultation between members of the staff of the service and other physicians is frequent.

An appraisal of the service was made by Professor Nellis B. Foster, of Cornell University, New York, on the medical side; by Professor Ransom S. Hooker, of the College of Physicians and Surgeons, New York, on the surgical side; and by Michael M. Davis, Ph.D., of the Julius Rosenwald Fund, Chicago, on the administrative and service side. These experts judged the service to be of excellent grade.

The service thus offered by the Endicott Johnson Corporation is a very heavy charge against the business, and could not be undertaken properly except by an industrial organization of great soundness and stability. On the other hand, it is quite possible to take the view that, in the long run, the heavy carrying charges for this service are in fact passed along to the consumer, and thus may be regarded as an indirect form of taxation. Viewed in this way, it is evidence of the possibility of delivering good and complete medical service to persons in the lower income brackets without employing either the principle of insurance or requiring a collection of funds through taxation.

THE HOMESTAKE MINE MEDICAL SERVICE [5]

This service is offered by the Homestake Mining Company, of Lead, South Dakota. This company is engaged in the mining of gold, and has a very assured and steady income. The service was instituted in 1910 to offer complete medical care to employees and their families. In 1930, the service cared for about 5,332 people. The care offered includes office consultation, home service, hospital service, and medicine. Eyeglasses are supplied at cost. No dental care is provided, nor any home nursing. The employees have freedom to choose their physicians from the members of the staff. The service is offered free of charge to the group above-mentioned.

The staff consists of five full-time physicians. These physicians are all primarily general practitioners, but some of them have devoted time to special fields and, therefore, are properly classified as partial specialists. They are not permitted to engage in private practice. Their salaries range from $3,000.00 to $10,000.00, with an average of $5,280.00. As in the case of the salaries paid by the Endicott Johnson Corporation, these are net incomes and, therefore, compare favorably with the average incomes of medical practitioners.

Cost.—The total cost, in 1930, was $79,325.63, or $14.88 per eligible person. The portion of the cost which should be allocated to industrial injury—that is to say coming under requirements of the Workmen's Compensation Act—was $10,630.00, or $1.99 per capita of employees.

It is of some interest to compare these per capita costs with the medical charges paid by other members of the same community to physicians in private practice. There is a basis of comparison here in a group of about 9,000 families not coming under the group cared for by the Homestake Medical Service. Study of this point develops the fact that for families with an income of from $1,200.00 to $2,000.00 the fees paid to private physicians are somewhat less, while families having an income of $2,000.00 to $3,000.00 pay somewhat more than the cost of the Homestake Medical Service. However, the family cared for by the Service gets about six times the number of office calls, and from 40 to 90 per cent more home calls than does the family employing private physicians. If the families cared for by the Medical Service had been charged the rate of fees customary among private physicians in this region, the expense to the Homestake Mine would have been $175,378.00, instead of $70,977.56. The service here offered is definitely less complete than that offered by the Endicott Johnson Corporation. The medical staff is smaller and less specialized. Yet, the service appears to represent a good grade of medical care. The physicians employed by the service are well satisfied. The recipients of the service continue to use it, though

88 GROUP HEALTH SERVICES

they are under no compulsion to do so. The views held by the physicians practicing in the neighborhood in regard to the character of the service vary as would naturally be expected. However, it is not reasonable to expect that they would wholly approve of it, nor is it reasonable to regard them as unprejudiced witnesses.

THE BOROUGH OF SWINDON [6]

Swindon is a town of 65,000 inhabitants in the county of Wiltshire, England. It has several independent factories and industrial establishments, but the main business is the local engineering works of the Great Western Railway. It is essentially a prosperous town. Half the population, for instance, own their own houses. The wages at the railway vary from £2 12s. 6d. (about $13.12 at par) to £8 10s. (about $42.50) per week. Few families earn less than £3 ($15.00) a week. There is very little poverty.

The Great Western Railway Medical Fund Society was organized in 1847, and has had a continuous successful existence. It is important to note that this was started before the passage of workmen's compensation laws, and sixty-five years before the passage of the National Insurance Act. It offers medical attendance, but no financial benefit.

Sources of funds.—Each member makes a weekly contribution. Since the passage of the National Insurance Act, "panel patients" pay the following scale: Single men, 3d. (six cents); married men, 6½d. (thirteen cents). Non-panel patients pay a somewhat larger amount: Single men, 5d. (ten cents), married men 8½d. (seventeen cents). The company makes some contribution toward capital expenses, and supplies fuel, gas, electric light for the premises of the Society, and makes repairs. It takes a part, though only a small one, in the management of the Society.

Service offered.—The services offered by the Medical Fund Society are dispensary care, home visits, hospital care, consultant care, and laboratory work.

Membership in the Society.—The Society had, in 1929, 17,000 members, who, with their dependents, constituted a group of 45,000 people—which amounts to about two-thirds of the population of Swindon.

The medical staff.—The medical staff consists of a medical superintendent, who is also the medical consultant. His salary is £1,400 (about $7,000.00). There is a consulting surgeon, who is also assistant medical superintendent, at the same salary. There are nine assistant medical officers, with salaries varying from £700 to £900 ($3,500.00 to $4,500.00). These officers are all on whole-time duty, except for the consulting surgeon who is allowed to have outside consultations and perform outside operations. There is a consulting röntgenologist and a consulting pathologist. There are four wholetime dental surgeons, at salaries varying from £450 to £800 ($2,250.00 to $4,000.00). The hospital has a matron and a nursing staff. The dispensary is open from 9:30 A.M. to 7:30 P.M., and dispensary visits can be so arranged that the men can attend without loss of working time. Home visits are arranged for in the morning, except in emergencies.

Volume of work.—In 1928, there were nearly 101,000 dispensary visits. For the purpose of home visits, the Swindon area is divided into nine districts, each with a separate medical officer. If an employee moves from one district to another, he will then come under the charge of another medical officer. It will be noted that there is here practically no freedom of choice, but the evidence appears to show that there is no dissatisfaction. If the patient desires another physician, it is arranged that he shall be seen by the physician in charge, with the consulting physician. If this does not work out satisfactorily, and he wishes to make a change in his physician, the proper arrangements are made.

Hospital treatment.—The hospital is lodged in a temporary building, having thirty-six beds. This equipment is not satisfactory, and further development is necessary. During the year 1930, 570 patients received hospital care.

Obstetrics (Midwifery).—The fund provides medical care in midwifery cases, but expects the member to book a duly qualified midwife, as is the custom throughout Great Britain. During the year 1930, 103 such cases were attended in the home, and 40 cases at the hospital.

The development at Swindon is important. It is an entirely voluntary plan offering relatively complete service with limited freedom of choice of physicians. During its more than eighty years of existence it has worked satisfactorily and has continued to operate equally well since the passage of the National Insurance Act. In fact, it supplements the service offered under the act in many important particulars. It differs from the two other examples of industrial medical service in that it is only in a minor degree a charge against the business. As in the other examples of industrial medicine, it is probably dependent for its satisfactory workings upon the presence of a relatively very stable and important industry.

COMMUNITY MEDICAL SERVICE

In many respects the examples of community medical service which will be discussed are quite similar in organization to those discussed under the heading of industrial medical service. They differ, however, in the essential fact that they offer service not only to people employed in the industry, but more or less to the whole community. For this reason it seems proper to discuss them under a separate heading.

COMMUNITY MEDICAL SERVICE AT ROANOKE RAPIDS, NORTH CAROLINA [7]

The service was organized by five industrial companies, and their employees. The companies were the Roanoke Mills Company, the Rosemary Manufacturing Company, the Patterson Mills Company, the Halifax Paper Company, and the Virginia Electric and Power Company. Somewhat later, an arrangement was made by which the teachers, and a small group of nurses, were included with the employees of these companies. This makes a total of 4,919 people. The organization offers medical service to the employees, as above defined, and their dependents. It also offers the same medical service to other residents of the city and county.

Service offered.—The service offered includes hospital care, office visits, home calls, and laboratory work. The offering does not include dentistry, drugs, medicines, or expert care in diseases of the ear, nose, and throat.

Funds.—The corporations pay the salaries of the physicians and of the visiting nurses. They also pay certain fixed charges at the hospital. The employees contribute twenty-five cents a week, which is deducted from the payroll. A small group of 130 teachers pay $25.00 a year, and a still smaller group of 13 nurses pay $24.00 a year. The other residents of the community, who desire the service, pay on a regular fee-for-service basis. The average weekly wage, of both the mill and the non-mill families, is $17.50. The average weekly family income of the mill employees is $24.50, while the average family income of non-mill employees is $27.16.

Medical staff.—The medical staff consists of five physicians and three visiting nurses. The average net income of the physicians in 1930 was $8,409.00.

Cost.—In 1930, the total cost of operation was $226,264.00. Of this sum, what may be described as the organized service—that is to say, the service for which the organization pays—cost $147,536.00, 65.2 per cent of the total expenditure. The cost of the non-organized service, which includes drugs and medicines, dentists, and special ear, nose, and throat care, special nursing, was $78,728.00, or 34.8 per cent of the total expense. The per capita cost to the mill people was $17.63. There is clear evidence that, if this service had been purchased in the regular, unorganized way, it would have cost about 35 per cent more.

From this brief sketch, it is clear that the service offered at Roanoke Rapids is definitely incomplete. Also, it is not managed wholly on a contributory basis, since a considerable part of the income is obtained on the ordinary fee-for-service basis. Like all other medical services centering about industrial establishments, its security will be definitely influenced by business conditions. However, taking into consideration the fact that medical service in southern mill towns is often quite incomplete and quite unsatisfactory, this organization clearly offers relatively assured medical facilities, and a considerable proportion of its financing is done directly by contributions from the payroll. It also has the very definite advantage that there is no middleman involved in the supplying of this care, and that there is no insurance carrier involved.

FORT BENNING MEDICAL SERVICE [8]

An interesting example of organized community service is to be found at Fort Benning, Georgia. Fort Benning is a military post, but it is also the Infantry School of the Army. This tends to give it a stable, and relatively high income-bracket population. In this respect it differs importantly from the medical services offered to industrial groups. In 1930, the number of people entitled to care was 7,790. Of these, 46 per cent may be classed as family groups—that is to say, officers and their dependents, other ranks and their dependents, and servants, who are regarded as the dependents of the officers. They may also be divided as follows: officers and other ranks, 5,283, dependents, 2,507.

Medical organization.—The medical organization was set up for the purpose of providing complete medical care, without cost to the group. The staff consists of a Station Surgeon with the rank of colonel, seventeen medical officers, four dentists, nineteen nurses, 148 enlisted men (orderlies, technicians, laboratory assistants), three lay administrative officers, and fourteen civilian employees. The physical plant consists of a main hospital building and three ward buildings. These have a normal capacity of 191 beds, but can be expanded in emergency to 363. There is a laboratory building, a nurses' home, a main dispensary building, and four other dispensaries placed at convenient points. The whole setup might be likened to a medical center.

The medical staff.—The medical staff is so planned as to offer fully equipped general medical service, consulting service, and specialized service. It is a very complete organization, and is fully utilized.

Cost.—The cost in 1930 was $400,000.00. If all expenditures are included, this means a per capita cost of $50.67 a year. Divided into classes, the military group showed a per capita cost of $55.03, the dependent group, $41.48, and the family group, $45.54. If the fixed charges on the hospital establishment—that is to say, interest on capital investment, and depreciation on buildings—be deducted, the general per capita cost was $40.90. Comparing this with the surveys of family expenses at an income level of $3,000.00 to $7,000.00, we find that, the country over, the average expenditure of such families was $41.24. But, the group at Fort Benning got very much more service than is obtained by the general family groups of similar income the country over. In terms of office visits and home calls, they got more than three times the amount of service. It is interesting to note the extraordinary difference in the cost for drugs and medicines. The Fort Benning group spent $0.72 per capita, whereas families in the same income groups of the general population spent $4.86, which is nearly seven times as much. In regard to the cost of hospital illness, the figures are also interesting. At Fort Benning the cost per case was $48.06. In representative family groups from the general population, those in the income group of less than $1,200.00 spent, on the average, $67.38 per hospital case, and in the income group at $10,000.00, or more, the cost per hospital case was $468.62.

Salaries of the medical staff.—The medical staff are all officers of the Medical Corps of the Army of the United States. The average salary of the group was higher than the average income of physicians in the United States, but it was lower than the income of physicians whose training and experience would make them comparable. It should, however, always be remembered that these members of the various medical services of the United States have at their backs the assurance of a pension. This is an item by no means negligible for those who are approaching the height of their physical activities.

Quality of the service.—It will not be necessary to do more than point out that the quality of the service rendered to the group at Fort Benning is of thoroughly first-class calibre. Not only can this be attested to by many witnesses, but it was, in fact, the expressed opinion of Professors David Riesman and George P. Muller, of the University of Pennsylvania.[9]

VII

THE WORKMEN'S COMPENSATION ACTS

Legislation for workmen's compensation, commonly referred to as the Workmen's Compensation Acts, is the direct result of an evolutionary process resulting from the changes taking place in industry as the result of the Industrial Revolution. With the first development of industry, even though it was not at all comparable to present conditions, the old common law relation between master and servant rapidly disappeared. In the earlier days such a relationship was reasonable, and operated satisfactorily, but with the growth of industrial establishments such a relationship became quite impossible, since the master, in the majority of the cases, did not even know the servant by sight. However, out of this relation of master and servant there grew up three basic principles in the common law which served as defences in litigation brought against the employer, for injury. The first was the doctrine of "fellow servant" under which it was held that where injury resulted from the fault of a fellow servant, the employer could not be held liable. The second defence was the doctrine of "the assumption of risk," under which it was held that an employee assumed the risks of the occupation. Finally, there was the doctrine of "contributory negligence," under which the employee was required to show that the accident was not the result of his own carelessness. As a result of these defences it commonly was impossible for an injured employee to recover in the courts.

As this situation became evident, various countries took cognizance of the fact, and laws were passed removing these defences and making the employer legally liable for financial compensation. The legislation resulting in Employer's Liability came more slowly in this country than in England, where it was established in 1880. In the United States, the first legislation on this subject was in Massachusetts, in 1886, following rather closely the British law, and, during the subsequent twenty years, most of the states passed similar legislation. It is important to observe that these laws concerned themselves particularly with questions of financial liability and were not at all concerned with questions of medical care. Even under these statutes the position of the employee was far from satisfactory. No one, who was familiar with the multitude of tort cases which literally choked the law courts in industrial regions, could fail to be struck by the great advantage possessed by the employer. In the first place, he was commonly represented by expert counsel employed by the liability insurance companies, which appeared in this country first in 1886, and offered to employers insurance against liability. Under this insurance, the company provided the legal talent, collected the necessary witnesses, and was prepared almost from the time of the accident to put every obstacle known to the law in the way of the injured employee. On the other side may be cited the tendency of juries to sympathize with the employee, even though the case against the employer was weak, and, on the whole, to award rather large damages, on rather insufficient evidence. The whole atmosphere was that of a legal game in which the power of the corporations was pitted against the employee, even though the latter was often able to find very expert lawyers to plead his cause. As has so often been the case, the real question at issue, namely, the propriety of protecting the employee from injury received in the course of his work, was quite forgotten, and the performance became a gladiatorial contest between legal experts, aided and abetted by medical experts, often frankly partisan to the people who hired them.

The Workmen's Compensation Acts

Out of this unsatisfactory, if not unsavory, situation arose the compensation acts. They are referred to in the plural since they are statutes of the individual states, passed at different periods, and varying importantly in their specific provisions. Between the years 1911 and 1920, Workmen's Compensation Acts were passed in rapid succession by many states. Forty-four states, the District of Columbia, and three territories had enacted such legislation by 1930.

It will be evident that in the brief space at our disposal it will be impossible to discuss the intricacies of these acts, and only a general outline of their common principles will be possible. It is important, however, in order to understand the apparent difficulties which these acts have encountered, to appreciate that at the outset they were frankly intended to supply compensation for injury, and that, particularly in the earlier acts, little or no thought was given to the important part which medical care would inevitably play. Thus, many of the earlier acts gave only the most cursory consideration to the provision of medical care, and it seems often to have been regarded as a rather unimportant side issue. It is perhaps for this reason that the medical profession showed very little interest in the development of this legislation, and rather early found itself at a disadvantage in pointing out the inadequacy of the provisions for medical care.

FORM OF ADMINISTRATION

Practically all the acts are administered by a state commission, though in some instances a single commissioner is substituted. These commissioners, obviously are likely to be, and in fact generally are, political appointees, and often hold office only at the discretion of the appointing power. This has tended to weaken the administration of the acts, since permanency of tenure, which would be so valuable, is commonly lacking. Some states authorize the insurance carriers to be of four types: (1) insurance stock companies, (2) mutual companies, (3) self-insurance by financially sound corporations, and (4) special state funds. Under the various statutes, these state funds either may be exclusive, which means that the insurance is carried by the state alone, or competitive, in which case the state insurance fund is in competition with stock and mutual companies. The rates for insurance carried by the stock and mutual companies are established with the approval of the state commission, and subject to adjustment. Commonly, the stock companies are allowed about 40 per cent of their total receipts for overhead expenses, while the mutual companies are allowed about 20 per cent. Competitive state funds commonly allow about 10 per cent for these purposes, while the exclusive state funds spend only about 4 per cent. Thus, it is evident that the amount of money allowed for overhead expense to the stock company is relatively large as compared to the amount actually spent either by competitive state funds or, particularly, by exclusive state funds. This amount is entirely lost for the purposes of compensation and payment for medical care, though the companies

THE WORKMEN'S COMPENSATION ACTS

insist that it is not more than is necessary for the handling of the business. It may be noted, in passing, that in Canada all of the funds are under exclusive provincial management.

GENERAL PROVISIONS OF THE ACTS

These acts provide compensation for injury. There is generally a waiting period of short duration during which no compensation is paid, and a limit of amount and of time. They also provide payment for medical care, though in some of the earlier acts this provision was omitted. The amount allowed for medical care was, in the earlier acts, obviously inadequate, and has been continually raised. The most characteristic thing about both of these types of compensation is that they have been the subject of constant disagreement and constant amendment. There has been, on the whole, a steady increase in the amount of compensation for injury and in the amount of coverage for medical care. Today, the latter is almost unlimited in most states, as far as legal provisions are concerned. In 1931, at least $72,000,000.00 was paid out under the provisions of these acts for medical care.

It is important to realize that the overwhelming majority of accidents come within the waiting period, so that in only a small percentage of the cases is any cash compensation paid for time lost. In 1920 only 2.85 per cent of the injured employees received compensation for time lost, while in 1930 this had diminished to 1.55 per cent. On the other hand, of the 98.45 per cent who received no compensation for time lost, a large number, undoubtedly a large majority, received medical care, often amounting only to first aid. How important this waiting period is, in cost to the insurance fund, is shown by the fact that when, in the state of New York, the waiting period was diminished from fourteen to seven days the payments for compensation increased by a million dollars. In order to make more clear the importance of the proper arrangements for medical care the following figures are quoted. In 1931 it was estimated "that there were 90,000,000 industrial injuries in the United States annually, of which only 3,000,000 are of sufficient severity to require cash compensation." [1] The same observer estimated that the average cost in the 87,000,000 temporary injuries was $2.00 each.[2]

DEFINITION OF INJURY AND ACCIDENT

These conditions are ordinarily defined in the acts, but the physician commonly has grave difficulty in making them fit the classification. On the face of it, it would seem as if these questions were, or should be, purely medical, since they appear to require expert judgment in the medical field. Curiously enough, however, the commissions, composed of laymen, have constituted themselves medical experts, and in this they have had the support of the courts. Thus the Supreme Court of Wisconsin said:

In this case the trial judge apparently accorded the testimony of these physicians full faith and value. But it does not follow that the Industrial Commission attached any such weight to their testimony nor do we think they were bound to do so. If the testimony of these witnesses was contrary to their own expert knowledge upon the subject, they were at liberty to disregard it.[3]

The California Industrial Accident Commission, in 1927, said:

For many years it has been the unchanging opinion of the medical profession that hernias are not of traumatic origin in the sense that they are rarely the result of a single strain or injury, but, rather, are caused by the successive strains to which the physical body is subjected in the ordinary course of living. Within the last two years the Commission, with its experience acquired in this field, reached the conclusion that the medical profession was not entirely correct in its position on this question.[4]

That trained experts of the medical profession should find it at times difficult to reconcile such legal and lay opinions with the well-tested evidence of science is not surprising. It is just this sort of tendency to disregard the testimony of experts, and to rely upon the highly fallible judgment of political commissioners, that has given rise to so much disagreement in the carrying out of the acts and has, on the whole, seriously interfered with their greatest usefulness. On the other hand, it is proper to note that the medical profession is not without blame for this situation. In the earlier days of the development of these compensation acts, it held almost wholly aloof, and either was frankly not interested or was likely to be found in opposition. This point is important, since if any further development is to take place in the scope of these acts, and particularly if other legislation is to be expected covering the development of insurance in questions of health, the medical profession should learn a lesson from its failure, in the past, to inform itself sufficiently and to offer its expert advice at the appropriate time. That further extension of the scope of these acts is probable, may be judged from the fact that there is already a distinct tendency in state legislatures to extend coverage to include occupational disease. Should this be done, a very much more comprehensive system would be developed, and one in which the importance of medical care would be even greater.

SELECTION OF PHYSICIANS

As a rule, under the acts, the insurance carriers are allowed to select the physicians who shall care for injuries. The stock companies commonly select physicians, or groups of physicians, to care for injuries in the industries which they insure. The mutual companies have often set up elaborate, and quite complete, hospital establishments. The industries which insure themselves may set up a medical organization at the plant, and have often done so. Such an organization may vary from the employment of a part-time physician assisted by a trained nurse and perhaps an orderly, to provision for very complete medical care employing several full-time medical experts. This question of the selection of physicians has given rise to a never-ending discussion between the medical profession and the insurance carriers. It is probably true that much of this discussion might have been avoided if the medical profession had taken a more active part in the planning of legislation. At the present time, the recasting of legislation has become an increasingly difficult business. The contention of the carriers is that, since they are required to pay for the medical care, they have a right to select physicians who in their judgment were capable of doing the work. The medical profession argues for freedom of choice, and the war goes merrily on. Curiously enough, a pretty good case can be made on either side of the argument. Thus, the insurance carriers feel that when the employee is allowed to select his own physician, he is likely to select one who is not competent to care for the particular condition, and, furthermore, that the selection having been made, the importance of the injury is likely to be magnified in the interests of increased compensation both for the physician and for the employee. On the other side, it is said, with perhaps equal justice, that the physician selected by the insurance company will be biased in favor of returning the employee to his occupation within the waiting period or, at least, within the shortest period which is conceivably possible. As evidence of the position taken by the medical profession, one may quote from the publication of the International Medical Association.

One of the principal factors in a cure is mutual confidence between the patient and his doctor. This implies free choice of the doctor by the patient. The Association therefore demands, as an essential condition of the satisfactory working of the medical service in sickness insurance, that freedom of choice be guaranteed by the legislation of all countries.[5]

The Bureau of Medical Economics of the American Medical Association comments upon this as follows: "Advocates of social change cannot afford to flaunt so unanimous an opinion as those who may be presumed best qualified to judge the facts on which that opinion is based." One may be pardoned for suggesting that the opinion of the International Medical Association is to some extent a prejudiced one, and for hesitating to regard the medical profession as the best qualified group of experts to pass upon so complicated a question as freedom of choice.

In support of the view that selection of physicians by the employer or insurer is on the whole a sounder method one may quote from a decision of the Connecticut Board of Compensation Commissioners.

On the whole, an average higher grade of medical, surgical, and hospital service is, in my opinion, secured under the Connecticut Act under which the employer or the insured has the right to designate the surgeon, than would be secured if the employee selected his own surgeon. Both humanity and enlightened self-interest require that the insurer and employer select from the most skilled and reputable physicians and surgeons of the community, and this was true in the case at bar, and is generally the case; but if these cases cannot be handled in such a manner as to inspire confidence on the part of workmen, some modification of the present system may naturally be looked for in the course of time.[6]

It would be possible to continue to quote such conflicting opinions almost indefinitely. The extraordinary divergence, and the fierceness with which each side defends its opinion, tends to show that there is probably something to be said upon both sides. It appears to me obvious that there is danger that the employee will not have the knowledge requisite to select the most competent physician available, and that he will be in some danger of selecting a relatively incompetent physician who he believes will act in such a way as to guarantee him the largest amount of disability compensation. This is, after all, but a natural reaction of human nature under circumstances where all of the elements necessary to a wise choice are not available. On the other hand, there is convincing evidence to the effect that the insurance carriers are likely to select physicians whom they can employ at relatively low compensation, and who will tend to act in their interest. If these conclusions are correct, it appears to me to follow that the selection of physicians by either party is open to objection. However, it may be argued that, after thorough conference between the commission and the authorized representatives of the medical profession, a system could be worked out under which the medical profession would undertake to supply the commission with a list of thoroughly qualified experts, from which list the employee would be required to choose. This, of course, would put upon the medical profession a requirement to police itself, and would go quite beyond any responsibility which it has hitherto assumed. On the other hand, it appears to me implicit in the situation that, unless the medical profession is prepared to make such selections and to assume full responsibility for the capacity of the physicians selected, the public which ultimately pays the bill cannot be expected to be satisfied.

PAYMENT FOR MEDICAL SERVICES

The satisfactory adjustment of scales of payment for medical services has yet to be achieved. That payments are on a more satisfactory basis is quite certain, but this improved situation has been arrived at only by a constant succession of more or less acrimonious discussions. It is important to recognize at the outset that it is in the regulation of payments for medical service that the carriers can make their profit. The amount which the carrier may receive from industry is generally fixed. The amount which he may charge to overhead and carrying expenses is also commonly fixed. It thus happens that the extent to which he can hold payments for medical care to a low rate represents his possibility of making a profit. This undesirable situation came about in the earlier days of the acts, when the amount allowed for medical care commonly was written into the law. Frequently, these allowances were ridiculously low, and, almost universally, they have been increased. But, even at the present time, the amounts allowed for medical care in most states are below that for which first-class medical care can with certainty be obtained. As the situation now stands with the stock companies, the proportion of the dollar expended for various purposes is roughly as follows: Of each dollar "approximately 42 cents goes to the carrier, 38 cents is spent for cash compensation, and 20 cents is spent for medical and hospital services." On their side, however, the carriers put forward the argument that when the compensation was not accurately fixed many physicians have been in the habit of padding their bills in the expectation that, after a considerable reduction was demanded, they would still receive a satisfactory fee. The fundamental difficulty, in arriving at the proper figure, is that there is no satisfactory standard. If the standard set be that of the fees ordinarily charged for similar work in that particular community, it will appear very difficult to determine what is the average charge for similar work, since the medical profession is still operating under a sliding scale of fees which vary within very wide limits.

PAYMENTS TO HOSPITALS

In some respects, the case of the hospitals is worse than that of the physicians. Thus, if the above basis be used in fixing charges, it at once appears that many of the patients seeking care under such conditions are likely to be indigent, and the hospital may receive nothing for their care. In practice, it is quite clear that the hospitals of the country have on the whole lost large amounts of money, often essential to their proper management, as a result of the workings of the acts. On the whole, however, the situation in regard to payment for medical services has steadily improved, and in many or most states it is now upon a reasonable basis. In the year 1929, it seems probable that something in the neighborhood of $77,000,000.00 was paid for medical services.[7] This is a very large sum, and would compare favorably with the amount of money expended in most countries having compulsory health insurance, with the probable exception of Germany.

RELATION OF THE MEDICAL PROFESSION TO THE COMPENSATION ACTS

That the relation of the profession, as a whole, to these acts has been unsatisfactory is one of the most obvious things about the operation of the acts. As already suggested, part of the difficulty has arisen because of the profession's lack of interest during the period of development. But, part of it has certainly come about because doctors proverbially dislike to be bound by rules not of their own making, and are much in the habit of doing things their own way. From the beginning the medical profession has objected to what may be called the "paper work." Under all of the acts a considerable number of reports, often required at definitely stated periods, and sometimes in considerable detail, is necessary. The objection of the profession has not always been well-advised, since it is inherent in such legislation that, since the responsibility for payment is through a third party, this third party must have the necessary data. No physician is under any compulsion to do any work under the compensation acts, but if he undertakes to do so, he cannot properly object to the regulations laid down by the proper authorities.

On the other hand, many or perhaps most of the commissions are so constituted that they are without satisfactory medical advisers of their own, and are constantly facing questions requiring expert medical opinion. That their decisions are often at variance with accepted medical opinion is therefore not surprising. My reading of the record brings me to the conclusion that, as a rule, the compensation boards, or commissions, are made up of reasonable people. They have generally shown a willingness to consider medical advice coming to them from the proper sources. The best results, I think, have always been obtained where the medical profession deals with the commission through the medium of a properly organized and relatively stable committee. The extent to which the relation between the commission and the profession improves is almost directly in proportion to the willingness of the profession to set up satisfactory means of intercommunication, and to give time to the constant adjustment of disputes and disagreements. The unsatisfactory working of many of the acts has been an excellent illustration of the fact that the medical profession has not thought it worthwhile to set up a proper organization and deal with the whole problem as one of public interest. Where such arrangements have been made and carried out, the results have been reflected directly in improved relations. It is perhaps true that the state of Ohio is the best example of satisfactory organization on both sides. At any rate, great improvement has resulted from a coöperative, helpful, and public-spirited attitude on the part of the medical societies. Much, however, remains to be done in improving the relation of the medical profession to the compensation laws. There is still evidence, on the part of the profession, of an uncoöperative attitude. There is still evidence, on their part, of a lack of conviction that this method of dealing with the casualties of industry is here to stay. They have failed, on the whole, to face their entire responsibility as public servants to an extent which would have made the acts more workable and more satisfactory to all concerned. I do not enter, at this time, into a discussion of the lines of development which may be desirable for the future, but it is proper to point out here that these acts, which have grown up without much assistance from the medical profession, are a very long step toward the participation of the public in the care of accident, injury, and disease developing in industry. There are probably more people today included under these acts than are included under any of the compulsory health insurance systems of other countries, with the possible exception of Germany. We have here before us an outstanding example of the extent to which legislation may run ahead of expert knowledge and may build up precedent and conditions on the whole undesirable, which might have been avoided had the doctors been alive to their full responsibility as public servants.

Contract Practice [8]

Contract practice has been defined by the Judicial Council of the American Medical Association as follows:

By the term "contract practice," as applied to medicine, is meant the carrying out of an agreement between a physician or group of physicians as principals or agents and a corporation, organization or individual, to furnish partial or full medical services to a group or class of individuals for a definite sum or for a fixed rate per capita.[9]

This is a very broad definition, and covers a great variety of conditions which actually exist, today, in this country. As a matter of fact, contract practice in one form or another is of very ancient origin. It is barely possible that the medicine which, it is alleged, was practiced in China many centuries ago, by which the physician undertook to keep the patient well, constitutes the beginning of such practice. In more recent times, fraternal orders, trade unions, and similar organizations have executed contracts for various types of medical care. The contract practice with which we are now chiefly concerned was much stimulated by the passage, by the various states, of Workmen's Compensation Acts. (The states of Arkansas, Florida, Mississippi, and South Carolina have no Workmen's Compensation Acts.) The contract practice which has grown up in connection with these acts is closely related to various types of industrial medicine previously discussed, but as it constitutes a common method of dealing with medical problems of industry in certain parts of the country, it requires fuller discussion. It developed chiefly out of the requirement to provide medical care of the type prescribed by the compensation acts, and, also, out of the necessity of providing medical care for ordinary sickness to groups of workmen, and their families, in more or less isolated communities. It has been particularly important in the lumbering and mining industries. Except in the states above mentioned, employers in these industries are required to provide care for injury occurring during employment. The provision of this care makes it desirable and proper that parallel arrangements should be made for the care of the health of employees not covered by the requirement of the law. In 1930 there are said to have been 540,000 men, employed in the lumber and mining industries, whose health requirements were more or less covered, outside of the requirements of the compensation acts, by a deduction made from the pay roll.

The problem of railroad employees has had to be handled on a different basis, since, as they are engaged in interstate commerce, they do not come under the requirements of the state compensation acts. In 1930 there were about 530,000 railroad men, thus engaged, for whom provision had to be made. Though there is no federal workmen's compensation act, men employed in interstate commerce have some protection under the Federal Liability Law, which is similar to those liability laws of the various states, which preceded the enactment of the Workmen's Compensation Acts. In general terms the railroad men are looked after, in respect to injury, by funds, part of which are contributed by the road, but a larger part by the employees. In the case of many of the roads, the associations which handle these funds automatically include in their membership everyone employed by the road. Most of the railroads have a system of company surgeons widely scattered in the territory served by the railroads, whose business it is to give first aid and care to injured persons, whether employees or passengers. Hospital care is arranged for separate from the funds, sometimes in company-owned and -operated hospitals, and sometimes in "designated" hospitals. As a rule, the company pays for the care of injuries sustained while on duty, and also pays compensation for time lost. This plan has been worked out by agreements between the railroads and their employees. Some roads have very elaborate hospital systems. Practically all the roads have a chief surgeon, generally a full-time salaried officer, and many company surgeons, sometimes on a part-time salary, and sometimes on a fee-for-service basis. The companies also provide these surgeons with "passes" on the road. In the case of railroads which own and operate hospitals, this department is ordinarily separate from the arrangements with the company surgeons. Frequently, some of the surgeons of these hospitals are on full-time salaries; sometimes, all of them are. The more common arrangement is to have a surgeon in charge of the hospital on salary, and the surgeons associated with him on a part-time basis.

Contract practice, as developed under the stimulus of the Workmen's Compensation Acts, has a distinctly regional distribution, chiefly due to the industries employing men in isolated and thinly populated areas.

WASHINGTON AND OREGON

In these states, contract practice has developed to a large extent. The compensation laws allow the employer to contract with physicians, hospitals, or hospital associations, for the care of industrial injuries. They are also allowed to make deductions from the pay roll for the medical care of non-industrial accident and illness.

Washington.—In this state, there are two general plans under which such arrangements may be made. The so-called "State Plan" provides for a fund made up of contributions from employer and employee, known as the State Medical Aid Fund. Under this plan the workman chooses his own doctor or hospital, and payment is made from the fund. The employer furnishes transportation to hospital or physician, where required. The other plan is the co-called "Contract Plan." An employer, with the consent of 50 per cent of his employees, may contract with a physician or hospital for the care of industrial injuries. Under this plan, 10 per cent of the contributions are paid to the State Medical Aid Fund, and 90 per cent is paid directly to the physician or hospital. All such arrangements are subject to the supervision of the Industrial Insurance Commission. The "Contract Plan" applies only to compensation cases, but the system has been much extended, by coöperative arrangements, to cover non-compensation cases. The two contracts thus arranged for are planned to give "complete coverage."

In order to make the matter clearer, a typical case may be cited. Under this the employer agrees to deduct ten cents a day from the pay roll, up to a maximum of one dollar a month. Of this sum, 90 per cent is paid to the contractor, whether a physician, hospital, or hospital association, on the fifteenth of each month. The contractor agrees to furnish all necessary medical, surgical, and hospital care for the employee and his dependents, both for compensation cases and for other injury and illness. It is stated that the bulk of the medical work is done by a relatively small number of hospital associations and clinics. Nevertheless, there are also many individual physicians who have individual contracts with corporations. This type of contract is largely employed in the lumber business, but has also been extended to other fields. During the last few years the contract system has extended rather rapidly.

Oregon.—The Workmen's Compensation Act provides for an Industrial Accident Fund, made up of contributions from employers and employees. The employee contributes one cent per working day, and apparently, on the average, the contribution of the employee is about 15 per cent, while that of the employer is 85 per cent. It is further stipulated that the total contribution may vary from 2 to 5 per cent of the pay roll according to the hazard of the business. From this fund the Industrial Accident Commission pays cash compensation, medical care, and transportation. There is also an arrangement allowing for contracts, which may be either between the Industrial Accident Commission, or an employer, and an incorporated hospital association or physicians. All of these contracts are under the supervision of the Industrial Accident Commission. There may be two separate contracts: one, with the State Commission for Industrial Accidents, and a separate contract covering non-industrial injuries and illness. The law specifically forbids profits or rebates.

CALIFORNIA

The Workmen's Compensation Act passed in 1911 required the employer to provide medical care for industrial accidents, at his own expense. It left the employer and employees free to arrange for care for non-compensation cases. These arrangements are supervised by the Industrial Accident Commission. This law was amended in 1917 to provide for supervision of hospitals and hospital funds by the requirement of an annual report to the Commission which should show the amount collected or received, expenditures, and the balance. For non-compensation cases, it is the custom to make pay roll deductions varying from $0.50 for a single man, to $1.80 for married men. It is stated that, in 1930, 49,483 employees, chiefly in the lumber and mining operations, participated in group plans providing compensation for non-industrial accidents and ordinary sickness.

THE ROCKY MOUNTAIN STATES

These include Idaho, Montana, Nevada, Arizona, New Mexico, Utah, and Colorado. All of these states have Workmen's Compensation Acts. In Idaho, Montana, Nevada, Arizona, and New Mexico, the employer must provide medical care for injuries covered by the compensation acts, but may make pay roll deductions, not to exceed one dollar a month, for medical and hospital service in non-compensation cases and ordinary sickness. In Colorado and Utah it is provided that there shall be no charge for compensation cases, but that deduction from the pay roll may be made for medical care of other kinds of sickness, and that the charge shall be commensurate with the service. In practice the results are about the same, the men getting medical and hospital care, the payment for which is divided between the employer and employee.

Coal mining.—In 1930, there were said to be 25,768 men employed in this work. In Wyoming medical care is provided jointly by contributions from employer and employee as part of annual wage agreements. A so-called hospital commission is set up at each camp, with three members—one representing the company and non-union employees, and two representing the union. These commissions receive and disburse funds, and enter into contracts with surgeons and hospitals.

Colorado.—The Colorado Iron and Fuel Company maintains a relatively elaborate service. This provides full medical care, with company hospitals and full-time surgeons. A physical examination is required on employment, for which one dollar is charged. The service is maintained by a fund contributed to by the company, and also by pay roll deductions. A separate fee is ordinarily charged for non-compensation hospital cases.

The other companies, as a rule, employ a company physician, on salary. Pay roll deductions are made for the care of non-compensation injuries and ordinary sickness, which includes the care of the family. As a rule, these companies do not own or operate hospitals.

Utah.—In this state, the companies ordinarily have a contract with a physician, and make pay roll deductions for care not coming under the compensation acts. These deductions vary from $1.00 to $2.50 a month.

CENTRAL STATES

These include Michigan, Illinois, Indiana, Iowa, Kansas, Missouri, Oklahoma, and Arkansas. In Michigan, Illinois, and Indiana, it is not customary to employ company doctors except for the care of cases coming under the compensation act. In Illinois some of the local unions have made medical arrangements, but this is uncommon, and there is no connection with the company. In Iowa, Kansas, Missouri, Oklahoma, and Arkansas, there is no general system of company physicians. In a number of instances there are miners' hospital associations. These are wholly operated by employees. The company collects funds by a checkoff from the pay roll. In these employees' associations a contract is entered into with a physician. Membership in the association is ordinarily placed at five dollars, with a monthly charge of one dollar. This provides medical care for the employee, and his family, in non-compensation cases.

Arkansas.—This state has no Workmen's Compensation Act. In the bauxite industry, there is a company hospital and company physician. A pay roll deduction of $1.00 for single men and $1.50 for married men is made. This does not cover the cost of service.

THE LAKE SUPERIOR IRON MINING INDUSTRY

This is located in Michigan and Minnesota. There is commonly a company medical service, which supplies medical care both for compensation and non-compensation cases. The usual pay roll deduction is $1.25. These companies are ordinarily self-insured. In Minnesota a company may be self-insured by obtaining a license from the Industrial Commission, which entitles it to make pay roll deductions for medical care not coming under the compensation act. The commission carries out an inspection to ascertain that the service is commensurate with the charge. These licenses run for one year. Many of the mining companies own and operate hospitals, and employ physicians on a contract basis.

MICHIGAN COPPER MINING FIELD

In the Michigan copper mining field, in which, in 1929, the Calumet and Hecla Consolidated Copper Company was the most important company, medical and nursing service is ordinarily provided, with a pay roll deduction of $1.50, to cover the cases not coming under the compensation act.

THE APPALACHIAN COAL FIELD

This is situated in the states of Pennsylvania, Maryland, Ohio, West Virginia, Virginia, Kentucky, Tennessee, and Alabama. In 1929 there were said to be 368,933 men employed.

Pennsylvania.—The anthracite coal industry is situated chiefly in northern Pennsylvania. In this industry, there are no deductions from wages for injury or illness not coming under the compensation act, and it need not, therefore, be further considered.

In the bituminous industry there is commonly a fixed deduction from the pay roll, and a company physician. This arrangement provides for office care and home visits. Generally no hospital service is provided. Two companies own and operate their own hospitals, making a pay roll deduction from $1.00 for single men to $1.75 for married men. These hospitals are staffed by capable physicians.

Ohio.—The common plan here is that of the company physician, with a pay roll deduction. Some of the companies have set up funds from which is supplied fairly complete service.

West Virginia.—The common arrangement in this state is that of the company physician, and a pay roll deduction of $1.00 to $2.00. There is a separate arrangement for hospital care, with an additional pay roll deduction of $1.00 to $1.35.

Virginia.—There is apparently here no uniformity of method. There is commonly a company physician, who may be paid on a fee or salary basis. The pay roll deductions for this service vary from $0.50 to $1.50. Three large companies have arranged for insurance, and have put up bonds with the Industrial Commission. They own and operate their own hospitals. There is a pay roll deduction for home and office visits, varying from $0.90 to $1.80. Hospital care is charged extra, the charge per case varying from $5.00 to $30.00.

Kentucky.—The common system in this state is that of the company physician, with a pay roll deduction of $1.00 to $2.00. In the eastern field, which is the largest, hospital care is generally provided. In the western field it is generally not provided. Two large companies in the eastern field own and operate Class A hospitals. These constitute instances of well-developed industrial medicine.

Tennessee.—The common system in this state is that of a physician employed by the miners, with a pay roll deduction of $1.00 to $1.50.

Alabama.—The common system in this state is that of the company physician, with the furnishing of medical and hospital care. Often there are two separate pay roll deductions: one, to cover office and home visits; the other, to cover hospital care. The Tennessee Coal and Iron Company has a very complete system. In 1931, it employed approximately 20,000 men, of whom about 4,000 were coal miners. Of the employees, 73 per cent were negroes. The whole group, with their families, constituted about 90,000 persons. The company owns and operates a 320-bed general hospital, 20 dispensaries, and emergency hospitals. It employs 73 full-time physicians. The expense of this establishment is borne partly by the company (45 per cent), and partly by the men (55 per cent). There is a pay roll deduction of $1.25, for office and home visits for the men and their dependents, and a hospital charge for non-compensation cases of $1.25 a day.

THE HOSPITAL CONTRACT SYSTEM IN THE WEST VIRGINIA COAL FIELD

This system exists chiefly in southern West Virginia. It has grown up because the Workmen's Compensation Act of that state is, to put it mildly, unclear. The difficulty arises because deductions from the pay roll to cover injuries coming under the act are not clearly, specifically, and entirely forbidden. Under this system, the company contracts with a private hospital to care for all illness, both compensation and non-compensation cases, except obstetrics and venereal disease. These hospitals are privately owned and operated for profit. There is ordinarily a pay roll deduction covering the care by the company physicians, and also a pay roll deduction covering hospital care. These deductions vary from $1.00 to $2.00. There is no requirement that the care of compensation and non-compensation cases shall be entirely separate. It is obviously to the financial advantage of these privately owned, profit-making hospitals to provide the least possible care which will give reasonably satisfactory results. There has been much complaint. The system grew up because, in the isolated communities in which these mines are operated, hospital facilities ordinarily were not to be found. The weakness of the law permitted the organization of these hospitals for profit and the system has been widely used. The fault appears to be due primarily to the law. An attempt to amend the law in 1931 failed. In states in which the wording of the law is entirely clear this difficulty does not appear to have arisen.

VIII

THE INCOME OF PHYSICIANS

In 1929 there were about 142,000 physicians in the United States engaged in the active practice of medicine. Of this number, approximately 21,000 were believed to be in full-time salaried positions. It therefore appears that, on that date, there were in the neighborhood of 121,000 physicians in private practice. Several studies have been made to determine the income of physicians. All of these surveys must deal, of necessity, with a section of the total group physicians, but, taking them separately and together, it is believed that they offer a reasonably accurate estimate of such incomes.

Physicians in Private Practice

It might appear that the selection of the year, 1929, is not calculated to give a fair estimate. It was certainly a year of relatively great prosperity, quite the equal of the two or three previous years, and certainly better than any subsequent time. The selection of this year will give a favorable view, and while it may be admitted that this picture may be unduly favorable, it certainly cannot be argued that it shows a situation less favorable than we shall have reason to expect in the immediate future.

Taking these various estimates together, it is a reasonable assumption that the average gross income of physicians was in the neighborhood of $9,020.00, while their average net income was in the neighborhood of $5,304.00.[1] For our purposes, it is not essential that these estimates should be regarded as strictly accurate, and it is certainly safe to assume that the average gross income of physicians, in that year, was somewhere between $8,000.00 and $10,000.00. This, on the face of it, would appear to be a pretty satisfactory average income, since there are not over 3 per cent of the population who earn as much. On this basis the total gross income of physicians in that year was in the neighborhood of $1,090,000,000.00—which means about $9.00 per capita of the population.

If we inquire into the way in which this average gross income is distributed among the profession, we shall find the following. Forty per cent went to physicians who were complete specialists, 22 per cent went to physicians who confined their practice partly to a specialty, while only 38 per cent went to physicians engaged in general practice. It is engaging to study how this gross income is distributed among physicians, according to the localities in which they practice. Thus, in towns and cities with a population of under 5,000—which contained 48 per cent of the population of the country—there were 30 per cent of the physicians, who received only 18 per cent of the gross income.

We may next inquire concerning the amount and distribution of net income. The spread between gross and net income for physicians in private practice is large. This is accounted for by the relatively expensive equipment which, even in the case of the general practitioner, is considerable, and, in the case of the specialists, may amount to a very large item. In this overhead expense is not included the cost of purchase or operation of automobiles. As has been said, the average net income of physicians in private practice in the United States was, in 1929, about $5,304.00. This may be compared with the figures on income of the general population, which would classify physicians with the upper 5 per cent of the incomes of the country. But these net incomes are very unequally distributed. Fifty per cent of the physicians receive not more than $3,800.00, 25 per cent receive not more than $2,300.00, 15 per cent receive not more than $1,500.00, while 4 per cent showed an actual deficit. In other words, at the end of the year they were worse off than at the beginning.

Put in another way, 50 per cent of the physicians received only 17 per cent of the total, while 10 per cent received 36 per cent of the total. From still another angle, for every physician who had a net income of $10,000.00 there were two who netted less than $2,500.00.[2]

The relation of the income of physicians to the size of the community may be of interest. In communities with a population of less than five thousand, the median gross income of physicians was $4,372.00, while the net was $2,500.00. In cities with a population of ten thousand to twenty-five thousand, the median gross income was $8,574.00, and the net $5,150.00. In cities with a population of twenty-five to fifty thousand, the median gross income was $9,308.00, and the net $5,600.00, while in the cities with a population of from five hundred thousand to a million, the median gross income was $8,303.00, and the net $5,200.00.[3] It is interesting to note, from the above figures, that the incomes of physicians appeared to be higher and reach their best level in cities of from twenty-five to fifty thousand inhabitants. In general, it may be said that the income of the physician is at its lowest in rural communities, in which half the physicians receive less than $2,500.00 net income. This is a really serious situation.

The contrast between the income of general practitioners and specialists, to which allusion has already been made, is striking. In general terms, the average gross income of complete specialists was 150 per cent higher than the average gross income of general practitioners. In somewhat more detail, the average gross income of the specialist was $16,304.00, and his net income $10,000.00, while the average gross income of the general practitioner was $6,421.00 and his average net income $3,900.00.[4] Though the point has already been discussed, it may be worth while to repeat that it seems a fair estimate to place the proportion of specialists to the total number of physicians in private practice at roughly 40 per cent.

As collectors of their fees, physicians make a rather poor showing. This may be interpreted in various ways. One is inclined to regard it as evidence of a carry-over from their historical background, which makes the business aspects of practice notoriously uncongenial. Many of us can remember the time when it was not regarded as quite suited to the dignity of the physician to send any bills at all. Another possible interpretation is, that in his concern with the treatment of the sick, the physician has failed to accomplish a satisfactory adjustment to the principles and practices of a thoroughly commercialized world. Whatever may be the cause, the fact is clear. In general terms, in 1929, physicians collected only 81.5 per cent of their charges. This is really a shockingly bad showing, as compared with business collections. At that time, the average bad debts of manufacturing corporations are reported to have been 0.4 per cent. The bad debts of a group of amusements, hotels, and similar enterprises, was only 0.5; the average for all business was less than 0.6. As compared with this, in another somewhat similar group, Leven estimates that the uncollectible bills of dentists probably do not average more than 2 or 3 per cent.[5] But, even here, the general practitioner comes off worse than the specialist. On the average, the general practitioner collected only 79.7 per cent of his charges, while the specialists collected 84.1 per cent.[6] Moreover, collections get worse as incomes get lower. The general practitioner with a gross income of less than $2,000.00 collected only 57.7 per cent of his charges, while the specialist with an income in the neighborhood of $3,000.00 collected only 60 per cent. Rising in the scale, the general practitioner with an income in the higher brackets, between $4,000.00 and $5,000.00, collected 76.5 per cent of his income, while his colleague in a specialty, with an income between $3,000.00 and $10,000.00, collected 80.5 per cent. Thus, it is clearly evident that the income of physicians is not high, that for the general practitioner it is low, and that the relatively large incomes accumulated from the practice of medicine go to a very few individuals.

To make matters still more unsatisfactory, the working life of the physician is short as compared with that in most other occupations. At the present time, he is not likely to enter active practice until he is about twenty-eight years old. At that age, his expectancy of life is only thirty-nine years. If, after a wearing life, he should look forward to retiring at about the age of sixty, he will have at his disposal only thirty-two years in which to pay off any debts which he may have accumulated for his education, develop his practice, and leave at his disposal something with which to take care of his family and his old age. Now, in these thirty-two years which he may be thought to have at his disposal, the earlier ones will show relatively low earnings. It is estimated that he will not reach his median earning capacity for about seven years, during half of which period he will earn less than $4,000.00, gross. His income will probably reach its peak in the seventeenth or eighteenth year of his practice, and begin to decline, so that after he has been in practice about thirty-five years, it will have receded to the same figure, roughly, as in the seventh year of his practice.[7] If these figures are studied in connection with his net earnings during that period, the conclusion can hardly be avoided that, on the present basis of the private practice of medicine in free and open competition, the returns are not such as to raise great enthusiasm from the point of view of cash return.

Income of Salaried Physicians

The number of physicians whose income is on a salary basis is relatively small, and, consequently, statistical data drawn therefrom are likely to be less accurate. Moreover, it is difficult to define the group, since there is a considerable number of physicians on part-time salaries, in whose income these salaries play an important rôle, and there is also a considerable number of physicians, indicated as being on full-time salaries, who still increase their income by a certain amount of private practice. The group is neither large nor clearly defined. In 1929, there were estimated to be about 21,000 physicians on full-time salaries.[8] Of these, the average median net income was $4,213.00, as compared with an average median net income for private practitioners of $3,705.00.[9] Of these salaried physicians, 10.2 per cent had a net income of some $2,000.00 to $3,000.00, as compared with 16.2 per cent of private practitioners. Those with an income from $3,000.00 to $4,000.00 were 33.6 per cent, as compared with 12.5 per cent of private practitioners. Those with an income between $4,000.00 and $5,000.00 were 24.3 per cent, as compared with 9.5 per cent of general practitioners, while those with an income of from $5,000.00 to $6,000.00 were 15 per cent, as compared with 7.7 per cent of private practitioners. Dealing with cumulative percentages: 13.2 per cent of salaried physicians had an income below $3,000.00, while 40.7 per cent of private practitioners were at this level; 46.8 per cent of salaried physicians had an income below $4,000.00, while 53.2 per cent of private practitioners were at this level; 71.1 per cent of salaried physicians were below $5,000.00, while private practitioners showed only 62.7 per cent; 86.1 per cent of salaried physicians were below $6,000.00, while 70.4 per cent of private practitioners were below this level; 92.4 per cent of salaried physicians were below $7,000.00, while 75.8 per cent of private practitioners were at this level.[10] This appears to show that the physicians in salaried positions have a much smaller percentage of very low incomes, and a very much smaller percentage of very high incomes. Practically 58 per cent of

TABLE III

DISTRIBUTION OF PHYSICIANS' PROFESSIONAL NET INCOMES IN 1929

INCOME CLASS	PERCENTAGE OF PHYSICIANS IN EACH INCOME CLASS		PERCENTAGE OF PHYSICIANS IN EACH INCOME CLASS AND IN ALL PRECEDING CLASSES (CUMULATIVE)	
	PRIVATE PRACTITIONERS	SALARIED PHYSICIANS	PRIVATE PRACTITIONERS	SALARIED PHYSICIANS
Less than $2,000	24.5	3.0	24.5	3.0
$2,000-$2,999	16.2	10.2	40.7	13.2
$3,000-$3,999	12.5	33.6	53.2	46.8
$4,000-$4,999	9.5	24.3	62.7	71.1
$5,000-$5,999	7.7	15.0	70.4	86.1
$6,000-$6,999	5.4	6.3	75.8	92.4
$7,000 or more	24.2	7.6	100.0	100.0
Median Income	$3,705	$4,213		

the salaried physicians have a net income between $3,000.00 and $5,000.00, while in private practice only 20 per cent are in this group. As would perhaps be expected, physicians on a salary are further from starvation and further from opulence, but nearer safety.

PROFESSIONAL FEES IN PRIVATE PRACTICE

Though the whole problem of the adjustment of medical service to the changed and changing condition of society is beset with many difficulties and intricate problems, there is none which is more difficult and more puzzling than the problem of professional fees in the private practice of medicine. It is probably beyond the capacity of any individual to state the problem clearly, and in such a way that any solution agreeable to the parties concerned is likely to result. Against this, may be set the fact that fees are one of the most difficult problems of the physician, that they may bring about grave misunderstandings between patient and physician, and that they, at times, put the physician in a most difficult ethical position. Thus, although I appreciate the difficulties of making any clear statement, I am convinced that some statement must be made.

Part of the confusion, which is evident in many discussions of the subject, comes from an attempt to deal with professional fees as if they had always been upon their present basis. The fact is that we have removed them from their original setting, and thereby quite lost our perspective. The so-called learned professions originated from the church, and with the church the professions of teaching, law, and medicine were for a long period closely associated. In fact, it is within the memory of men still living when the support of the minister and the doctor in substantial American communities was clearly regarded as a responsibility of the community. I can well remember general practitioners whose compensation was partly in cash and partly in kind, who were expected to supervise the health of the entire community, and did so, who lived safely upon the assumption that the community would provide for their support. They were not in the habit of rendering bills. The more well-to-do members of the community paid them in cash; the less well-to-do, in kind; and the more or less indigent, or shiftless, not at all. In fact, it is only within this century that it has been a regular habit of the physician to render bills after a business fashion. In New England, certainly, the older practitioners in my day rarely rendered bills, and almost never sent them more than once. This was a survival of the tradition of an earlier day. Within this century, and increasingly during the last fifteen years, the medical profession has been trying to accommodate itself to a thoroughly commercial setting which, if it is to maintain its position as a profession, it is bound to find thoroughly uncongenial.

The legal profession has been to some extent assisted by the fact that it is at times at least dealing with questions that have perfectly definite financial value. In the case of the settlement of estates, as an example, there has grown up a custom as to the relation between the value of the estate and the charges made by the legal advisers. This extends to a good many other transactions in which the legal profession is involved and, to that extent, has made their problems less difficult. On the other hand, to the extent that the legal profession is still dealing with individual private clients, to that extent their difficulties are similar to, although not identical with, those of the medical profession.

It is probably a mistake on our part to look to any other groups, for much assistance in unravelling this complicated problem, since there is not, and never will be, any other group whose problems are precisely the same. No other group has to deal with problems of so great importance and involving such high stakes. Upon the shoulders of no other group falls the burden of the decision of such problems: occasionally, those of life and death; frequently, those of health and happiness; and always of vital concern in enabling the individual to maintain his position in an active world. I insist, therefore, that we shall not get at the root of this matter by trying to follow the practice of any other existing group.

In theory at least, the fee of the physician is a charge for service, but any attempt to define the value of this service verges upon the impossible. Obviously, the value is intangible, unfixed—perhaps unfixable. When faced with problems of life and death, the individual will obviously obligate himself to pay anything, even though it may land him in the poorhouse. But, it by no means follows that this is any appropriate gauge of the fee which should be charged. To set any fixed value upon a given professional service, as, for instance, a surgical operation, requires that consideration be given not only to the circumstances of the patient, but to the gravity of the condition, the skill and experience of the surgeon, and the extent to which his professional reputation may be jeopardized, perhaps unfairly, by the outcome of his efforts. It is thus evident that fee for service cannot possibly be made to fit into the setting of modern commercial price-making, since it lacks the fundamental elements upon which such determinations must be based.

"The sliding scale" applied to medical charges had its origin, as above indicated, in days when medical practice was very different from what it is today. Furthermore, the physician was much more likely to be familiar with the circumstances of the patient, and the spread between maximum and minimum charges was likely to be relatively much less. At the earlier period, specialization was in its infancy, and the great majority of physicians were general practitioners who undertook to cover the whole field. The rapid development of specialization, particularly during the last twenty-five years, has immensely complicated the problem. The spread between the charges appropriate to general practice, and those appropriate to some of the more intricate and highly developed specialties has become enormous. The fact of the matter is that the development of surgery in its various divisions has, more than any other special development, complicated the question of professional fees. While it may be true that the extreme disparity between the fee of the general practitioner and that of the specialist is out of proportion to the value of the services rendered, it is beyond question that the services which are, or may be, rendered by the specialist have a spectacular character which appeals to the imagination and can therefore be made to command a relatively high price. Though the novelty of the surgical specialties has begun to wear off, their appeal to the imagination still remains. It is not difficult to think back to the day when an afterwards distinguished general surgeon, faced with the problem of a patient who had inadvertently swallowed his false teeth, boldly, and for the first time in medical annals, opened the abdomen, incised the stomach, removed the teeth, closed the wound, and the patient "lived happily ever afterwards." It is necessary to bear in mind that the services of the specialist may take on the appearance of life-saving measures more often than any services likely to be offered by the general practitioner. In general, it is true that the tendency to be critical of medical fees applies more frequently to the charges of the specialist than to those of the general practitioner. The establishment of fee tables by medical societies has not served a very useful purpose, since they can at best only suggest the average fees which may properly be charged under average conditions to the patient in average circumstances. Obviously, they are likely to be wholly inapplicable to almost every individual circumstance. It has been suggested that the fees, particularly of specialists, should be based upon the income of the patient and should represent a definite proportion of that income. This does offer some tangible basis for the estimate, and it has been suggested that for "capital" operations a charge equal to 10 per cent of the patient's income might be appropriate. While this might supply some basis for judgment, it of necessity leaves out of account all the peculiar conditions surrounding individual cases. Furthermore the development of the practice of installment buying, particularly in the last fifteen years, has given rise to a situation in which, though a patient may have a relatively fixed and satisfactory income, it may be wholly mortgaged in advance. Under these conditions to propose to the patient a fee equal to 10 per cent of his income, though it may represent a fair charge, may be entirely beyond his capacity to pay. As time has gone on and the situation has become increasingly complicated, there undoubtedly has arisen a tendency to that reprehensible practice, formerly charged against the great railroad systems, of putting the charge at what the traffic will bear, a method which only renders confusion worse confounded.

Viewed from a distance, the fees of the professions in general, and particularly medical fees, have come to bear something of the aspect of a graduated income tax. As a probably unavoidable result of the community aspect of the earlier practice of medicine, physicians have always given a large amount of service free of charge. They give another considerable moiety of their time to the care of patients who can afford to pay them only what their services will actually cost. It has remained for the more opulent members of the community to make up, through the fees they pay their physicians, for that proportion of the physician's time which nets him nothing. To some extent, these richer individuals may be said to be contributing to charity, but though they may be wholly willing to do so, it sometimes occurs to them to suggest that they would prefer to select for themselves their objects of charity, rather than have them selected by medical advisers.

No solution of the problem is here advanced, but it may be suggested that some relief could be obtained from the irritation of the present system, if the communities will face more squarely their obligation to care for the indigent. Today, there will probably be no general dissent from the proposition that the care of the indigent is a proper charge against the community, and yet, in this country at least, there has been a very incomplete recognition of that obligation. It is true that the community, by providing hospitals supported by taxation and staffed by able physicians, has faced the problem of serious illness, but almost nowhere has the community recognized the fact that the services rendered by the physician should properly be regarded as part of the cost of this care.

Admittedly, the present difficulty has grown up out of a past in which no similar expenditures of time and skill were required. The present uneconomic situation has arisen by an imperceptible growth, which has made it quite out of keeping with modern conditions. As the matter stands, it would seem that until such time as the community is prepared to accept the view that the time and skill, at present donated by the physician to the care of the indigent, are a service which should properly be paid for at a reasonable rate, people are estopped from grumbling at the apparently disproportionate charges which must be made to those who can afford to pay.

But, while this aspect of private medical fees has been troublesome and annoying, there are other aspects of the question which promise to prove even more difficult and serious. Allusion has already been made to the gross disproportion between the fees paid to the general practitioner and those paid to the specialist. These fees must be judged, in the long run, to have been established in more or less consonance with public opinion, which agrees that the services of the specialist are worth the price which he charges. Under our system of licensure, all physicians are theoretically free and equal. There is nothing to prohibit the general practitioner from extending his services into any special field with which he may feel competent to deal, and in which he can persuade patients to accept his services. Thus, it comes about that there is a grave temptation for the general practitioner to undertake surgery beyond the limits of the minor fields, and, since his experience and breadth of knowledge are much less than those of the surgical specialist, he frequently finds himself faced with conditions difficult, unexpected, and beyond his capacity. It is important to note that the willingness of the patient to allow a practitioner to undertake special work cannot be based upon any sound estimate of his training or ability. It is a shot in the dark which may well have a tragic result. There is thereby placed upon the moral fibre of the general practitioner a strain which may well exceed the strength reasonably to be expected of human beings.

The fee for service arrangement also may bear heavily upon the strength of character of the specialist. At an earlier period, when most of the surgical operations undertaken were those urgently required in order to save life or limb—commonly referred to as "operations of necessity"—little question could arise in regard to the proper indications. But, in the last thirty years, surgery has advanced to a point where now the great majority of surgical operations are no longer "operations of necessity," but have become "operations of election," which may be defined as those which are undertaken, not as emergencies, not to save life or limb, but to correct abnormality, to relieve discomfort, to prolong life not immediately menaced, and, to an increasing extent, to correct real or alleged abnormality of function. From this shift in the indication for operation flows the necessary consequence that much of the surgery of today has become a matter, not of clear indication, but of judgment. At a time when the undertaking of a surgical operation was fraught with grave danger, ill-judged or unnecessary operations were rarely undertaken, because so to speak the price was too high. But that situation no longer exists. The actual risk to life of most surgical operations has become relatively small, and an error in surgical judgment is fraught with no such obvious and serious consequences. This has had the effect of throwing upon the surgical specialist a responsibility for careful investigation and the use of sound and disinterested judgment, which was quite nonexistent at an earlier day. It has also had the effect of making it increasingly desirable that the public should have some relatively accurate method of gauging the training, experience, and judgment of those who hold themselves out as specialists. No such method has been devised, and there is no effective curb upon physicians with insufficient training and, perhaps, weak moral fibre, but with the advantages of personality and approach which recommend them to patients—who must make their selection by the most haphazard methods. Under these conditions, it is perhaps not surprising that ill-judged or unnecessary operations occur. It is more surprising that they do not occur more frequently.

Fee-Splitting

There is still another misshapen offspring whose parents are the development of specialties, and the fee for professional services. His name is Fee-Splitting. This wholly reprehensible practice may be defined as a division between the general practitioner and the specialist—but without the knowledge and consent of the patient—of the fee received by the specialist, ostensibly for his services. It would be difficult to say just when this practice first began, but it obviously had its origin in the rapid growth of specialization, and was beginning to be fairly well recognized in this country as a dishonest practice as early as 1910. That it was a matter of serious importance in 1913 is shown by the fact that, at the organization of the American College of Surgeons in that year, it was thought essential to include, in the requirements for membership of this organization, the avoidance of fee-splitting, under any disguise. The practice probably began with the desire of a physician who was attempting to build up for himself a surgical practice, to stimulate its growth. A surgeon of weak moral fibre would offer to general practitioners, having patients requiring his surgical services, a proportion of the fee which he expected to charge. In its mildest form this might appear quite harmless, in that the surgeon having operated upon the patient of the general practitioner and being unfamiliar with his financial status, might suggest to the physician that he decide the proper charge and retain what might be called a rake-off. This practice had apparently become relatively serious by 1913, but forthwith changed its aspect to some extent because the acquiescent general practitioner soon came to see that he could bargain with various surgical specialists, and enter into arrangements with those who were most complaisant. Thus, there has developed an appalling situation, in which physicians in general practice come to regard themselves as having something to *sell* to the specialist who will allow them the largest commission. One can see, creeping into a profession dedicated to service, practices which are common and not thought reprehensible in a highly commercialized world. It would, in fact, be too much to expect of any group that they should universally resist the accepted practices of a commercial age, particularly when such practices redound to their financial advantage. What has happened is that the requirements of a professional code of ethics have met, in head-on collision, the accepted practices of a commercial age. It is to the credit of the profession that these dishonest practices have never met with anything but official disapproval. Medical organizations in every field have persistently and consistently denounced them as dishonest and inconsistent with professional integrity. The Colleges of

THE INCOME OF PHYSICIANS

Surgeons and of Physicians, the American Medical Association, and many state and county societies, have time and again voiced their complete disapproval. Nevertheless, this disapproval has been quite powerless to prevent the spread of the practice and, in one form or another, it is today very widely prevalent. Obviously, those bodies which supervise the ethical standing of physicians are placed in a most awkward position. There is much testimony concerning the frequency of fee-splitting, but, in order to put a stop to it, not testimony, but evidence is required. Any medical group which undertakes to discipline one of its members, and in that process injures his professional standing, must be prepared to prove its case in court, or take the consequences. The members may be convinced in their own minds of the moral obliquity of their colleague, but it is quite another matter to convince a jury. Fee-splitting, of necessity, is a transaction, or series of transactions, between individual physicians, of which no evidence which would stand the test of the courts can ordinarily be produced. No amount of official disapproval has been able to importantly influence it, and there is no reason to expect that it can do so.

It is frequently intimated that the practice, though existent, is uncommon, and to that extent unimportant. As proof one way or another is not to be had, the extent of the practice remains therefore a matter of opinion. However, some evidence upon this point may be obtained from a recent questionnaire sent to physicians in a large Middle-Western city, by a physician who was a member of the local medical society. This questionnaire, sent to physicians belonging to the medical society and, also, to physicians not belonging to the society, asked their opinion on many points. Among others, a question was asked in regard to fee-splitting. The question was worded: "What are your ideas about fee-splitting?" Of 87 members of the society answering the question, 48 were favorable, 35 were opposed, and 4 were doubtful. Of 103 physicians, not members of the society, 57 were in favor of fee-splitting, and 46 were opposed to it. Even though I have been well aware for many years that fee-splitting was very widely practiced, I confess to being shocked that any considerable number of physicians, licensed to practice, should commit themselves on paper to such a statement. I feel required, as the result of experience over a considerable portion of the country, to express the well-considered opinion that the practice is common, that, at least in certain sections of the country, it has profoundly influenced the practice of medicine, that it is not diminishing, and that it is increasing. The extent to which such a practice now appears to exist is, I think, incompatible with the continuance of a dignified position for the profession. It is a practice which the profession must either destroy, or which will destroy the profession.

Free and Open Competition

At this point, it is important to call attention to the fact that many of the difficulties which surround the question of medical fees arise wholly out of the fact that the private practice of medicine is carried on under a system of free and open competition. The severity of this competition was very much less at the earlier day when physicians were more widely scattered over the country, and when specialization had only begun to develop. With the tendency, previously noted, of physicians to congregate in centers of population so that the number of physicians per capita is importantly in excess of the average, this competition obviously becomes increasingly severe. There is not only the competition between general practitioners for the general practice of medicine, but there is competition between specialists in their own fields, and, as pointed out above, danger of this competition leading to highly objectionable and dishonest practices. One frequently finds in modern medical journals, and even incorporated in the by-laws of state societies, the term "unfair competition." This phrase is strangely reminiscent of its common use in trade disputes, and tends to show the danger that the profession may be forced into the use of trade practices which will importantly jeopardize its standing.

Many of us were brought up on the old economic saying that "competition is the life of trade." Competition was certainly of the essence in the earlier days of the capitalistic system. However, as organized society has advanced under the capitalistic system, it has become increasingly apparent that, even in trade, competition is by no means certain to be in the interests of the consumers, and in many fields has proved objectionable. At the present moment we are witnessing what almost looks like a revolution in our views in regard to competition in business, and there is widely held opinion to the effect that, in many fields, competition has served its purpose, and that various forms of supervised and controlled monopoly are indicated for the future. Thus, it appears that, even in trade, we are coming to have doubts as to the desirability of competition, and very grave doubts as to the propriety of allowing the continuance of free and open competition. The objections which have appeared in regard to free and open competition in trade obviously will be likely to operate even more severely in fields properly occupied by professions. By its very definition, the profession of medicine must be chiefly and vitally concerned with the offering of service. Free and open competition may well interfere with the satisfactory offering of such service. It is proper to go even further and to point out that, since the objections to competition center largely about its effect upon the consumer, these objections must tend to become more weighty in a profession which deals exclusively with human life. It is not easy to believe that free and untrammeled competition, leading as it has to the various devices which will assist the individual toward financial success, is a proper method under which to deal with those conditions of life and death which are utterly fundamental to the security of society. Obviously, the evils of competition which become objectionable in trade may well become fatal in the field of medical service. It is by no means easy to reconcile the ideals of a profession of service with the increasing severity of the competition under which the medical profession finds itself today.

In this dilemma, it seems proper to point out various methods by which the most objectionable features of free and open competition may be lessened. It seems quite certain that the worst of them, namely, the dishonest division of fees, is most likely to occur where physicians are acting as isolated individuals, and will be more difficult to carry out when physicians are associated together in groups where there is considerable risk that dishonest practices will be discovered. To this extent it is possible that the association of physicians in organized groups, or such loosely organized groups as those which develop about a hospital, will tend to minimize these practices, and, to this extent, will mitigate the evil. The difficulty with free and open competition is that it tends to divert the profession from its original basis, in which the competition was primarily based upon excellence of service and recognition flowing from that excellence. When competition, as is too often the case, not only in medicine, but in other professional fields, tends to become competition in terms of cash, then it will inevitably tend to take on the practices and habits of trade. To the extent, therefore, that profits in cash can be removed, to that extent will the maintenance of a professional attitude be assisted.

It has frequently been asserted that the increasing tendency of physicians to work upon a salary basis is objectionable because it tends to remove certain incentives. This assertion does not appear to be based upon sound premises. Most people, whether in business or profession, work upon a salary basis, and there is relatively little evidence to show that this has destroyed, or importantly limited, their usefulness. One need only point to the enormous number of individuals working in many fields of science commonly upon a salary relatively meagre as compared with their intellectual capacity, who have continued to show persistence, energy, and idealism quite the equal of that which exists, or has ever existed, in any professional group. The question certainly does not turn upon the efficacy of fixed compensation, but does turn upon the ethical and moral fibre of those concerned. It appears to me to be a distinct affront to a group which has struggled hard to maintain its professional status to suggest that its efforts are importantly stimulated by a mere cash nexus. From a material point of view, there are many physicians who will work to better advantage if they are not constantly worried over the condition of their bank account, and, with the security which a salary basis will give, they could devote themselves whole-heartedly to the human problems before them, uninfluenced by the possible effect which their advice may have upon their financial fortunes. It may be admitted readily that the complete abolishment of competition in medical practice, particularly if it took place in a violent or sudden manner, would be highly objectionable or even disastrous, but this is a very different thing from wholesale opposition to the growing tendency to handle the practice of medicine in ways similar to those which now obtain for a large proportion of the legal profession and an overwhelming majority of the engineering profession. In attempting to pass upon such questions, one cannot avoid being influenced by one's own experience. During the last thirty years my time has been about equally divided between the practice of medicine in free and open competition, and the practice of medicine on a fixed or salary basis. During that period, I have had occasion to see, and become familiar with, many others in somewhat similar situations. I cannot remember meeting anyone who had experience under both these conditions who did not believe, in his heart, that the medical service which he offered while entirely free from the temptation and worry of open competition was of as good, or better, character as that offered under the strains and stresses of competition. Certainly, in many instances in my experience, one could go much further, and say that many individuals will do their best work under conditions which free them from financial strain. Now, it is not intended to suggest that medical practice should be transferred to a salary basis, but it *is* intended to suggest that there is fundamental weakness in the argument that salary, in and of itself, affects unfavorably the service which the true physician will give to his patients.

IX

THE ABILITY TO PAY FOR ILLNESS

Although there is a widespread opinion to the effect that the present cost of medical care is high, the soundness of this view may be questioned if it should appear that a notable proportion of the money is spent in undesirable directions. There may be considerable waste and duplication, and some of the money expended is, as far as it affects health, practically poured down the sink—in the purchase of patent medicines, often for conditions which are purely imaginary. The employment of inexpert quasi-medical people to do things for which they are quite untrained is also uneconomical.

Perhaps it would be proper also to indicate the possibility that a careful survey of the present situation might lead to the conclusion that while the amount of money expended bears heavily on some individuals, particularly at certain times, the total amount is not large as compared with the total income of the country, not large as compared with the importance of having a really satisfactory health service, and not as large as it ought to be if the job is to be properly done. These points must be dealt with later. At the present moment, it is intended to deal in general terms with the important questions of cost and ability to pay. As it will be necessary to use a variety of figures drawn from various sources, it is admitted at the outset that it is clearly recognized that figures may readily lead to very faulty conclusions, that the figures given as of a particular date may differ importantly from those drawn from equally reliable sources at a somewhat different date, and that any argument which assumes the complete, or even substantial, accuracy of such figures in its premises may well come to faulty conclusions. All that can reasonably be expected of the figures which will be quoted is that they shall be taken from sources known to have exercised care and skill, that they shall be intended to indicate general tendencies rather than narrow and specific conclusions, and that they shall be sufficiently accurate to indicate the direction in which these tendencies are headed.

The Cost of Illness

In 1929 the people of the United States spent a total of $3,656,-000,000.00, or $30.08 per capita for medical care.

Of this amount, $2,885,790,000.00 represented the fees of patients, $509,500,000.00 was paid from tax funds, $180,710,000.00 was met through voluntary contributions and donations, and $79,000,000.00 was borne by industry.[1]

An estimate of similar expenditures for 1931 shows a total of $3,225,000,000.00, of which, $2,625,000,000.00 was paid by patients, $400,000,000.00 was paid by the government, $100,000,000.00 each, was contributed by philanthropy and industry.[2]

The relation of these amounts to the national income may be judged on the following basis: The national income in 1910 was estimated at $31,000,000,000.00, in 1928 at $89,000,000,000.00, while in 1930 it is estimated to have fallen to about $71,000,000,000.00.[3] The amount spent for medical care is not an excessive proportion of the total income, particularly when one takes into account the many things, which must be classified roughly as luxuries, for which people spend money freely and willingly. Thus, in boom times, we spent over $12,000,000,000.00—more than four times the amount spent for direct medical care—for passenger automobiles, noncommercial use of gasoline, tobacco, candy, cosmetics, soft drinks, toys, jewelry, and amusements. Most of these expenditures were made by persons of moderate means, for whom the expenses for medical and hospital care are most pressing.

The amount spent each year for tobacco alone is about twice the total gross income of all physicians. The amount spent on candy is more than twice that expended on civil hospitals, and that spent for cosmetics is about twice the expenditures for nursing.[4]

In quoting these figures, it is not at all intended to suggest that these expenditures are not proper, but it *is* intended to suggest that large sums of money are available for things which the public desires, and of which it approves. Therefore, we need not boggle too much over the total bill, if it can be shown that this is to be paid for a desired and desirable article, and that the money is available for the people involved when the bill comes in.

Gross figures, such as those quoted above, give us, on the whole, very little information that we can use, as they are total costs which give no evidence of their relation to individuals. A somewhat more accurate view may be obtained by seeing how incomes are distributed, and, consequently, where the money is.

INCOMES

An estimate of national income and its distribution in 1928, based upon a study of the incomes of twenty-nine million families compiled from the census, including about 2,286,000 households of one person, gives us the following figures: 14 per cent of these families, which average four and one-half persons, had an income of less than $1,000.00; 30.3 per cent had an income of $1,400.00 or less; 68.1 per cent had an income of $2,500.00 or less; while 90.8 per cent had an income of $5,000.00 or less—leaving only 9.2 per cent with family incomes of $5,000.00, and only 2.7 per cent with incomes over $10,000.00.[5] It thus appears that more than half the families (55.3 per cent) have an income at or below $2,000.00. But, while the average income per family in 1928 was $3,105.00, there were less than 25 per cent who reached that amount.

EXPENDITURES FOR MEDICAL CARE

An estimate of the expenditures of average urban families, having four or five members, for medical care in 1928 and 1929, is illuminating. Of these average families, those with an income of $1,000.00 spent, on the average, $50.00 for medical care. Those with an income of $1,500.00 spent $75.00. Those with an income of $2,000.00 spent $90.00, while those with an income of $3,000.00—below which would be found 75 per cent of the families of the country—spent $120.00.[6] Thus, it is quite evident that much the largest amount of money was spent by the family with a relatively large income, constituting a relatively small percentage of the population. But, again we are likely to be confused by this question of the average.

The setting aside of certain sums of money for expenditures which are relatively fixed and certain is one thing, and may be represented by such fixed charges as food, shelter, and clothing. On the other hand, to set aside sums of money for illness is something entirely different since illness is wholly unpredictable and bears quite unevenly upon different people, leaving one family, or group of families, quite unscathed, while landing a staggering blow upon another group in equal or less advantageous circumstances. Some notion of the inequality of distribution of this burden may be gathered from the result of a survey of 8,581 white families with known income studied for twelve consecutive months, during the years 1928 to 1931. In the group having an income of less than $1,200.00 there was an average medical expense of $49.17, but the distribution was very uneven. Eleven per cent of the families paid over 50 per cent of the bill. Three and one-half per cent of the families had charges of $250.00 or more. By dividing the total medical expenses into thirds, we get the interesting result that 80 per cent of the families bore one-third of the expense, 17 per cent bore another third, and 3½ per cent bore the final third. In other words, the unfortunate 3½ per cent, upon whom illness bore most heavily, paid as much as was paid by 80 per cent of the families.

In the income group between $3,000.00 and $5,000.00 half of the total bill was paid by 86 per cent of the families, while the remaining half was paid by 14 per cent. Now, while it is conceivable that the average family with an income of $1,200.00 might be able to squeeze out $49.17 a year, a bill of $250.00 or more might completely wreck their finances.[7]

A further interesting comparison is the following. Taking the population at large, only 57 persons out of every hundred incur any medical expense in the course of the year. Four per cent of the total number receive nothing but free care, 39 per cent receive no care and incur no charges, 37 per cent incur charges ranging from 50 cents to $20.00, 15 per cent have charges between $20.00 and $100.00, and 5 per cent have charges of $100.00 and more. A somewhat different reading of these same figures shows that over half of the total medical bill is paid for care received by only 5 per cent of the population.[8]

Some interesting studies have been made as to the extent to which people, sick with disabling illnesses, do not have or cannot afford the services of a physician. Of twelve surveys made with this in mind, the best showing was made by that undertaken at Framingham, Massachusetts, in which out of a total of 407 disabling illnesses, 81 per cent were attended by a physician, and only 19 per cent got along without a physician. The worst showing was in Rochester, New York, where in 798 such illnesses only 61 per cent were attended by a physician, while 39 per cent of the sick people were not. If, however, one moves from the town of Framingham into the neighboring rural districts, one finds that 53 per cent of those with disabling illnesses were without medical care. The largest and perhaps, therefore, the most representative of these studies was that made in Pennsylvania and West Virginia. It included 7,333 cases, of which 73 per cent had a physician and 27 per cent had none.[9] This at least suggests that a fair proportion of the people who have no medical expenditures in any given year show this interesting, though deceitful, freedom from doctors' bills because of inability to command the services of a physician. On the other hand, it is of course possible that a certain percentage of these people, though quite capable of employing a physician, do not do so for personal reasons which, except in the cases of diseases dangerous to the public health, is perhaps not a proper concern of the community.

In considering these figures, it is of course essential to remember that these charges, all of which were made for physicians, hospitals, or medical accessories, were subject to the sliding scale under which physicians moderate their bills very extensively, and even withhold them entirely, in the case of persons with small incomes, while in the case of persons with large incomes their charges are proportionately very much greater, and are intended, to some extent, to make up for that portion in which their services have been given at less than cost. Thus, in the study of 8,581 families the average charge to families with an income under $1,200.00 was $49.17, while the average charge, to families with an income of $10,000.00 and over, was more than ten times as great—being $503.19. But, again the distribution of amounts cannot be gathered from averages. In the income group under $1,200.00, 69 per cent paid $40.00 or less, while 4.8 per cent paid $500.00 or more. In the income group of $3,000.00 to $5,000.00, though the average payment was $137.92, 42.4 per

THE ABILITY TO PAY FOR ILLNESS

cent paid from $200.00 to $1,000.00; in the income group of $10,000.00 or over, while the average was $503.19, 58.1 per cent paid from $500.00 to $1,000.00 or over.[10] This simply further exemplifies the impossibility of dealing with such questions on basis of the average. For instance, one family in the group under $1,200.00 will on the average have to pay $1,000.00 or more, which is obvious nonsense, while in the group of $10,000.00 or over, 2.7 per cent of the families will pay less than $20.00. This sort of evidence, which could be multiplied considerably, appears to be sufficient to show that illness, in almost any of the family income groups comprising a large percentage of the population, may very easily run to a figure entirely beyond their means.

Now it is of course theoretically possible to arrive at a figure, for each income group, which would perhaps provide the essential medical care, if the incidence of illness were regular and predictable. Thus it is arguable, though perhaps not reasonable, that the average family with an income of under $1,200.00 might be able to squeeze out $50.00 a year for taxes. It might further be argued that such an amount of money spent on the preservation of the health of the family group was well worth the price, but obviously no such situation exists. Such a family may go on for some years without disabling illness, and without being forced to pay out anything like this sum for conditions which they, themselves, regard as important. This, of course, should not be taken to imply that such families may not have medical conditions which urgently require care; it is only assumed that they, on the basis of their wholly inaccurate knowledge, have come to that conclusion. However, it is quite beyond the bounds of probability that such families can be induced to set aside annually, in a savings bank or other appropriate repository, any such sum on the off-chance that when the overwhelming catastrophe arrived they might have it on hand. To do so would cripple their style. It is useless to argue that they ought to do so, and that due care and foresight demand such moderation. The fact of the matter is that we, all of us, buy that which looks attractive, and which has, or appears to have, some immediate utility, or to supply some real or fancied desire. Nobody wants to pay for a doctor, or for a dentist, and there is no reasonable probability that any large group in the community will proceed in a way so at variance with their ordinary habits. Therefore, we may as well at once abandon the assumption that, since illness is irregular and unpredictable, it can and, therefore, should be provided for by some system of installment buying—often miscalled insurance—or of setting aside the estimated sums. Not only will this not be done, but in a fair proportion of the cases when all the savings have been made, at the figure alleged to be sufficient, on the average, to cover the cost, all too frequently it will be found insufficient. It would only require a few such experiences to shake the determination of the most careful and sturdy characters.

The Incidence of Illness

There are other interesting considerations in estimating the way in which illness will fall upon individuals or family groups. Thus, while the death rate for women is definitely lower than that for men, they have a considerably higher disability from sickness. This was shown very clearly in a survey made by the Edison Electric Illuminating Company of Boston. In the course of a five year study, it appeared that the average worker lost just under nine days a year on account of illness, including accidents, and that the average illness per worker per year was 1.28. The male employees showed an average illness of 1.03, while the female employees showed an average of 2.30, or more than double.[11] Thus, to the extent that there are women members of a family gainfully employed, they will raise the incidence of illness importantly. The presence of children in a family is an important consideration since they are notoriously liable to the so-called "contagious diseases" of childhood. Of these, measles is the most common, showing an incidence of 3.8 per thousand; scarlet fever, an incidence of 1.77; and diphtheria, of 0.90.[12] Thus, it appears that the presence, number, and age of children in a family will considerably influence the incidence of illness.

Furthermore, it is important to realize that the service received in the different income brackets varies very widely, as do the total costs. Not only do the people in the lower income brackets fail to call for medical service, but they can afford decidedly less of it. In a study of 8,639 white families, in which the survey was made with unusual care, the following evidence developed. The families varied from the lower income bracket, under $1,200.00, to that of $10,000.00. The incidence of sickness for which assistance was asked increased from the lowest to the highest brackets by 39 per cent, but, interestingly enough, the rate of hospitalization increased by 87 per cent. Calls by physicians increased by 145 per cent. Dental care increased by 651 per cent. Examination of the eyes for glasses, or refractions, increased by 552 per cent. Health examinations increased 333 per cent. This means, of course, not that the people in the higher income brackets had more illness that needed care, but that their illness was more likely to receive attention. If we should assume, which would perhaps be reasonable, that the lower income brackets required the same amount of medical care as the higher brackets, we should at once be driven to the conclusion that there is an immense amount of medical care required, that is not received on account of inability to pay. Whichever way we turn, therefore, we find this intruding difficulty of ability to pay. The amount of service which is quite obviously desirable is not received, despite the efforts of state agencies, the beneficence of charity hospitals and clinics, and the enormous amount of service donated by physicians.

Some engaging inferences may be drawn from a study of 38,668 white persons, in 8,639 families with known income, carefully surveyed. Thus, the rate of illness per thousand in the income group under $1,200.00 was 802.5, while in that of $10,000.00, or over, it was 1,111.5. The hospitalization showed an incidence in the first group of 59.4; in the last group, of 98.0. Home, office, and clinic calls showed an incidence of 2,169.2 in the lowest group, and 5,321.0 in the highest group. There is always apparent a steady rise, in the incidence of illness and care required, from the lowest to the highest group—except in the number of hospital days. Here, though the number of cases hospitalized in the group under $1,200.00 showed a rate of 59.4 as compared with 79.3 in the salary group from $5,000.00 to $10,000.00, the number of hospital days in the lowest group showed an incidence of 1,368.7 as compared with 896.0, an enormous increase in hospital days—which apparently indicates that when hospitalization was obtained for these cases, they were very ill, perhaps from lack of proper early care, and required much longer hospital confinement.

It is possible to assume that the amount of medical service called for by people in the higher income brackets is in excess of that really required. They may call their physician frequently, and for insufficient reasons. Of this there is very little evidence, and it is on the whole more probable that even the families with ample means consult their physicians less than would be desirable, particularly for problems in the field of preventive medicine. The study of the care received by the Fort Benning group (see pages 92-93) bears on this point.

X

HEALTH INSURANCE IN CONTINENTAL EUROPE

Whatever may be thought to be the problems of this country in providing itself with a satisfactory health service, it is safe to assume that somewhat similar situations have arisen in other countries. It is therefore important to survey briefly the measures they have taken to meet these conditions, and make some estimate of the extent to which conditions in other countries have been sufficiently similar to our own to enable us to regard their methods as of value in meeting our own problems. There will be no dissent from the proposition that a knowledge of measures taken by other peoples is of importance to us, though it by no means follows that any of these measures will be found applicable to our situation.

A study of methods adopted in Europe shows that they have been quite varied and, what is more important, that they have practically always developed out of previously existing conditions. It is quite conceivable that it might be possible to show that, in any of the European countries, the methods which have been adopted to improve their health service have been so intimately connected with the existing social and economic conditions that their adoption could have been almost predicted in advance. Even if this be an unwarranted assumption, it seems quite certain that the measures, which have been taken, have sprung directly from situations which grew naturally as the result of their historical development and their environment. It will not be possible even to describe, much less discuss in detail, the systems which have been adopted abroad. Selection will therefore have to be made, and it is hoped that such selection will present the outstanding features of plans and systems which differ sufficiently, both in their origins and in their development, to give a fair picture of the principles involved. At the outset, it should be noted that in 1930 twenty-five countries, not all of them in Europe, had adopted some form of compulsory health insurance, while seventeen countries were using some form of voluntary health insurance on a scale sufficiently large to constitute important evidence in the discussion. Some of the countries included in the group having compulsory insurance also have considerable developments in voluntary insurance.[1]

THE NETHERLANDS

The Netherlands is a relatively flat country, a considerable portion of it lying below the level of the sea, in which canals form an important element in transportation. Agriculture plays an important part, though navigation and commerce employ large numbers of people. The population is about seven and a half million. There are 3,827 physicians—a proportion of about one to 2,000 of the population. The medical provision is chiefly in the form of voluntary and contributory insurance. These measures cover chiefly what is known as the medical benefit—that is to say the direct care of illness—relatively little of it is for sickness benefit, a contribution toward lost wages. The health administration of the country is under the Minister of Labor, Commerce, Industry, and Health. In 1902 there was set up a Central Council of Public Health, having a membership of seventy unpaid members. Commenting upon the large number of members Sir Arthur Newsholme suggests that there may be economy under such a system, but says, "It must, I think, unless skillfully managed, act as a clog on prompt and necessary official activities."[2]

The purpose of this council is to advise and assist the government in the management of health problems. Its president, a physician, is the director-general of public health service. Acting under him are five chief official inspectors, whose functions are supervision over local sanitation and medical service. One supervises medical practice, including the medical care of the poor and the control of infectious disease. Another supervises pharmacy, food, drugs, and water supplies. A third is inspector of housing. A fourth looks after the enforcement of the laws concerning the inspection of food. The fifth has supervision of the care of tuberculosis and venereal diseases. Under these chief inspectors work divisional inspectors in the various districts. Sir Arthur Newsholme expresses the opinion that the care of the indigent in the Netherlands is not very highly developed.

SICK FUNDS (CAISSES)

A very large proportion of the wage-earning population holds membership in some organization supplying medical care. They make their own arrangements with the particular society. These arrangements include, not only care of the type given by the general practitioner, but also hospital care. In connection with what was said above, in regard to the background of these developments, it is important to note that some of the organizations date back to the seventeenth century. In Delft, they were in existence as early as 1603, in connection with guilds, and continued to develop during that century. As will be seen elsewhere, many of the existing sickness funds in various countries have their origin in guild organizations or, at a later period, after the guild had disappeared, in various trade organizations. At the present time in the Netherlands there is a great variety of these sickness funds. They may be listed in six groups: (1) general societies with local branches; (2) sick fund companies which are on a commercial basis; (3) funds managed by the employer, somewhat similar to funds which exist at the present time in the United States; (4) benevolent funds concerned chiefly with people close to the line of destitution; (5) mutual benefit funds founded and carried on by the insured; (6) funds organized by physicians or groups of physicians.[3] In regard to this latter group, it is interesting to note that such funds may be initiated by a single physician practicing in a small community, so that, in effect, a proportion of his patients pay him on an installment and not on a fee-for-service basis.

All of these funds have upper limits, fixing the income above which members will not be accepted. These, of course, vary widely with different societies. The upper limit will perhaps be found in the neighborhood of 2,000 guilders—about $800, at par. In the same way, the contributions vary widely. A common contribution is about twelve cents a week for a family, though it may run up to something like twice that amount. Most of the funds include children, without extra payment. It is sometimes stipulated that a man may not join unless his wife becomes a member. Also the financial management of these funds varies considerably. In some, there is a fixed sum or tariff which the family pays to the physician. In others, the total amount may be divided among the physicians and the druggists, after a proper sum has been set aside for management. In general, there is no freedom of choice of physicians, except within the group of physicians employed by the particular fund. This may give a moderate freedom of choice, or none at all. The physician deals directly with the officers of the fund on all questions of compensation. In some of the funds, which have a very large membership, a limit is placed upon the number of patients a given physician may have upon his list; the maximum ordinarily is placed at 2,500.

Entirely separate from this voluntary provision for sickness is the question of industrial accident insurance. This is compulsory, and entirely at the expense of the employer.

HOSPITAL CARE

In the Netherlands the supply of hospital beds is in the ratio of about three per thousand of the population. This ratio, as will be seen, is somewhat below that of some of the other neighboring countries. Moreover, the distribution of hospitals is quite uneven, varying from less than one bed per thousand in some parts of the country to nearly five per thousand in other sections. Arrangements for hospital care on prepayment basis are made separately from those concerned with ordinary medical care. They may be made through the same funds, or quite independently. Hospital care here, as in most of the countries, provides various types of accommodation—such as single rooms, two-bed rooms, and general wards. The care of the indigent in hospitals is looked after by the municipalities, though not necessarily in municipal hospitals. In general, it may be said that the Netherlands has gone unusually far in providing general medical care, at relatively modest cost, for a large proportion of the population under entirely voluntary organization. It is apparently true that this care is not as complete or elaborate or as well articulated with hospital care and provision for the service of the specialists as has been obtained in other countries.

OBSTETRICS

Special note perhaps should be made of the arrangements for obstetrical care. This is very largely in the hands of midwives trained and supervised by the state. The number of midwives is limited to about 900, which provides one to 8,000 of the population. Taking the country as a whole, about 60 per cent of the confinements are attended wholly by midwives. The proportion varies very much in different parts of the country, so that in some communes the proportion thus attended may be as high as 83 per cent; in others, as low as 35 per cent. Here, as in other countries where midwives play an important part in obstetrical practice, they are not expected to care for complicated conditions, and are required to call a physician should complications arise. In case a midwife is attending an indigent patient, she may insist upon the presence of a physician under these circumstances.

DENMARK

Nowhere has the principle of voluntary insurance against sickness been carried on so satisfactorily as in Denmark. (In 1933, the voluntary system was made compulsory.) This is probably a true reflection of the character of the country and its people. It is a small country characterized by cleanliness and order, relatively little poverty, and a relatively even distribution of wealth. The population in 1925 was 3,434,555. More than half the population is rural, but, on the other hand, Copenhagen has a population of 587,150.[4] A high level of general education and long-standing habits of coöperation have contributed importantly to the success of their system of sickness insurance.

HEALTH ORGANIZATION

The oversight of health is under the National Board of Health, in the Ministry of the Interior. The president of the Board is a physician. Like practically all European officers concerned with health he holds a life appointment and is entitled to a pension. This Board has supervision of the whole medical personnel—physicians, midwives, and dentists—as well as supervision of hospitals. There are some seventy district medical officers attached to the Board. Of these, twenty-three are county officers. These officers work under county councils, which are elective, but it is important to note that the chairman of these councils is appointed by the King on recommendation of the National Board of Health, holds office for life, and is pensionable. These district medical officers are charged with the care of the indigent, including their hospital care.

HOSPITALS

Before describing the system of sickness insurance, it is important to understand Denmark's hospital provisions, which are unusually highly developed, there being about 9.3 beds per thousand of the population. (In the United States, the proportion of hospital beds was 8.1 per thousand, 1931.) In 1924 there were some 22,709 beds—14,932 in general hospitals, the balance in contagious, mental, skin, venereal, and in hospitals for tuberculosis [League of Nations' Year Book, 1925]. These hospitals are municipal or county institutions. This quite extraordinary number and development of tax-supported hospitals is due to the fact that in 1806 the King of Denmark issued an Order in Council requiring each of Denmark's seventeen counties to have one to three hospitals, according to local need.[5] It may fairly be doubted whether such a system has its equal anywhere else. These hospitals are largely supported by taxation, but also make charges to patients, graduated according to their means. The charges made to members of medical benefit societies are not more than half the regular charges. Thus, it has come about that the use of hospitals by all classes of the population is very large. The medical staffs of these hospitals are state officers sometimes on full-time, and sometimes on part-time. Their salaries appear to be excellent. This arrangement is an important and an interesting one since, of course, it has the effect of separating the physician in outside practice from his patient on entrance to the hospital. It is also important as showing that, in Denmark at least, very satisfactory hospital work can be carried out on a salary basis. Newsholme says:

It is noteworthy, furthermore, that the large use of hospitals by persons of all classes appears to be accepted by private medical practitioners as unobjectionable. There is evidently behind this position a great weight of irresistible public opinion, apparently concurred in by the medical profession.[6]

This hospital system has a considerable subsidy, out of tax funds, to help out the work of the insurance societies.

MEDICAL ORGANIZATION

In Denmark, there are 2,500 physicians, 1,178 midwives, and 650 dentists—a proportion of physicians to the population of one to 1,400. All of this medical personnel is trained in the medical school and hospital of Copenhagen. The medical course covers seven years, and something like half of the students take an additional period, of what we should call internship, in hospital. The cost of medical education under the state is low. The course for midwives is two years, and they attend a large proportion of the births.

The medical organization of the physicians is the Danish Medical Association, to which nearly all belong. This association deals directly with the state in fixing the salaries of hospital officers, and with the insurance societies in fixing the methods and rates of payment for care of patients outside of the hospital. There is thus set up a direct relation between the government and the insurance societies on the one hand, and the organization of the physicians on the other. All the testimony goes to show that the relations have been eminently satisfactory, a situation which by no means always, or even generally, has obtained in other countries.

SICKNESS INSURANCE IN DENMARK

Sickness insurance in Denmark developed from clubs formed by groups or trades, and grew up, much as it did in England, from a spirit of mutual helpfulness. In 1885 the government offered to the clubs government recognition which provided a government subsidy for the groups, reduced rates at communal hospitals, and ambulance service to convey physicians or midwives to sick patients, or to convey patients to the hospital. In return for this assistance, the societies had to accept some restriction of their field, oversight of their bookkeeping, and a minimum cash benefit for specified periods of illness. As a further development, government inspectors were appointed, and there was set up a Central Board for Sickness Insurance. Anybody with an income below 3,800 kroner (about $1,026) is eligible. The scale of payments to these insurance societies varies with income. Those in the high income brackets pay a relatively large amount. In 1928, about 65 per cent of the population over fifteen years of age was insured. The monthly payments range from 1.20 kroner per month to 6.50 kroner. (One krone is about twenty-seven cents at par.) The disability insurance is an obligatory supplement to the voluntary health insurance. For these contributions, the individual gets not only medical care but also a monetary benefit during illness. On this basis, since the largest number of members are in the lower payment groups, there commonly results a deficit which is made up, partly by the central government, and partly by the town.[7]

It should be noted that though the system of sickness insurance is called voluntary, this does not tell the whole story. There is no compulsion on any individual to belong to an insurance society. On the other hand, if he does not belong to a society, should he have the misfortune to be overtaken by illness when his finances were in such a state that he had to ask assistance from the town, he would suffer serious disabilities in loss of the right to vote, prohibition of the right to marry without the permission of the authorities, and loss of his annuity for old age, which is a regular provision for members of insurance societies. It will be observed that this constitutes a kind of left-handed compulsion and was required "in order not to weaken their consciousness toward their own duties."[8]

PAYMENT TO PHYSICIANS

The payments to physicians may be accomplished by a fixed fee per patient or a fee according to service. This is done under various Tarifs. These Tarifs are most commonly used in cities, but are not uniform. In Copenhagen the rate is 9 kroner per member and 19 kroner per family without regard to numbers. In Jutland, on the other hand, Tarif I provides for a fee of 11.70 kroner per member and 23.40 kroner per family. Tarif II usually provides for a fee of 3.36 kroner for office visits and 4.20 kroner for house calls, plus travelling expenses. These fees are increased 50 per cent between 6 P.M. and 8 A.M. Physicians doing work on this basis may also carry on private practice. On the whole, the income of physicians is satisfactory. The choice of physicians is limited to those employed by the particular society and may thus give no choice, or, as for instance in Copenhagen where the districts may have some ten to fifteen physicians, there is considerable choice.

Contracts for this service are made between the Association of Sickness Societies and the Danish Medical Association. In 1925 the total income of the insurance companies was 43,700,000 kroner ($11,799,000), composed as follows: premiums from members, 26,500,000 kroner; allowances from the state, 13,000,000 kroner; other receipts, such as interest, 4,200,000.[9] In that year the total expenditures were 41,200,000. Invalidity insurance has been compulsory, since 1920, between the ages of fourteen and forty years. This invalidity insurance is made up by contributions from the insured, the employer, and the municipalities. As already pointed out, old age insurance is universal for all members of insurance societies over the age of sixty-five, without contribution dating from 1923.[10]

MIDWIFERY

The training of midwives is compulsory, and is supplied by the state in a two-year course. About thirty midwives are received every year for training. A very large proportion of the births in Denmark are managed by midwives. As in other countries, they are not supposed to undertake complicated or difficult labor, and must call a consultant. Curiously enough, considering the very large hospital provision in Denmark, it is said that most of the births occur at home, with the exception of the complicated cases. Physicians ordinarily do not concern themselves with normal obstetrical practice. Under this system, the puerperal mortality is low.

GERMANY

Germany* was the first large country to establish compulsory sickness insurance. Some study of the workings of this plan is therefore essential to any estimate of the value of this method of supplying medical care, since it has here been longest in operation, and has had, therefore, the best opportunity to develop evidence of strength or weakness.

* Everything which is here said about Germany will be understood to be based upon the government and conditions previous to the recent revolutionary changes and the dictatorship of Hitler.

The population of Germany is about 63,500,000. Something like 61 per cent of the population is in the state of Prussia, which is much the largest of the various states making up the federation.

It is probably true that compulsory sickness insurance was undertaken by Bismarck, in 1883, largely as a political measure. This has, unfortunately, often been true of similar experiments in other countries. It is said that it was his hope in this way to weaken the growing power of the Social Democrats. Whatever may have been its purpose, it failed to stop the growth of this and similar groups, and was, in fact, the beginning of a widening program of social insurance in many fields. This was much extended after the fall of the Empire in November, 1918. The social program after the war included a large list of such policies as unemployment insurance, old age insurance, disability insurance—as well as sickness insurance. This very ambitious program, undertaken under difficult postwar financial conditions, made worse by the widespread economic depression of recent years, will probably supply valuable evidence as to the extent to which social insurance can be undertaken without threatening national bankruptcy.

Our concern here, however, is wholly with sickness insurance, though it is perhaps wise to bear in mind that the development of the insurance program in a broader field has perhaps handicapped the development of the health program. Prior to the institution of compulsory health insurance there were a relatively few voluntary, trade and fraternal organizations, of moderate scope, working within this field. But, for practical purposes, the field had to be organized and insurance societies (*Krankenkassen*) were set up under the Insurance Code, with general government supervision, but not under government control. In this way, they sprang up as Territorial Funds, centrally located with widespread branch organizations, as Trade Funds and, to a smaller extent, as Mutual (guild) Funds. In 1930, about 71 per cent of the insurance was in Territorial Funds, about 24 per cent in Trade Funds, and about 5 per cent in Mutual Funds.[11] In theory these organizations are managed by representatives of the employers and employees—the insured. In practice they have often ceased to be representative of the insured, and very frequently have become political organizations of considerable power. In recent years many of the political parties in Germany have had their own very powerful insurance societies. In this way, the whole problem of health insurance has developed very important political aspects. Frequently, the questions which vitally concerned the management of the actual care of the sick were decided on political, not on public health, grounds.

THE INSURED

Compulsory insurance applies to all industrial employees, salaried personnel, and domestic servants, with an income of less than 3,600 marks.[12] (One mark equals approximately twenty-four cents.) Beginning with an insured group that amounted to only 10 per cent of the population, by 1928 it included 33 per cent of the total population, 63 per cent of the occupied population, and 77 per cent of the wage-earning population.[13] In most of the insurance funds, the insurance covers dependent persons, and in this way something approaching 99 per cent of the dependents of the insured persons are covered.[14] Unlike some other systems, particularly the British, later to be discussed, the *Krankenkassen* offer complete care, including home and office visits, hospital care, and the service of specialists. The contributions are quite uniform, one-third being contributed by the employer, and two-thirds, by the employee—the insured. It is further specified that the contribution of the insured shall not exceed 7½ per cent of the basic wage.

MONEY BENEFIT

As well as providing medical care during illness, these funds also provide a disability benefit. In this way there is introduced the complication, relatively common in broad plans of compulsory insurance, of handicapping the provision of medical care, with the giving of a monetary benefit. The difficulty, which will be more fully discussed later, is that this arrangement places the physicians in a difficult dual position. It may be assumed that the physician's primary concern is with the health of the insured, but, since he must pass upon the question of whether the disability is partial or complete, and must assess the period over which the disability lasts, he necessarily finds himself in the position of being pressed, on the one hand by his patient to extend the period of disability, and on the other hand by the *Krankenkassen* to make the period as short as is reasonable.

OTHER FORMS OF MEDICAL BENEFIT

In addition to the compulsory insurance which is carried on by business corporations (*Krankenkassen*) the German states also provide care of the indigent, a contribution in aid of maternity, contributions for child welfare—including school health programs—provisions for the care of tuberculosis, and provisions for the care of venereal disease. The methods of administering these various benefits have become enormously complicated, since they may be under the supervision of the Reich, under the supervision of the separate states, under the supervision of cities, or under the supervision of the communes. In this way, the complications become such as to beggar description by a foreign commentator, and one gathers that they get considerably confused in practice. In the case of provision for tuberculosis—for instance—there are organizations under the state, under municipalities, and a considerable proportion of patients with tuberculosis come under the Insurance Funds, when it occurs in insured persons or their dependents. No further attempt will be made here to discuss this complicated organization, since we are chiefly concerned with the organization and operation of compulsory health insurance.

HOSPITALS

In general, the hospitals in Germany, as in most continental countries, are chiefly constructed and operated by the government, but there are also many hospital establishments which have been built and are operated by the *Krankenkassen*. There are a considerable number of private hospitals. In 1927 there appear to have been 2,964 public hospitals, with 314,019 beds, and 833 private hospitals, with 44,310 beds.[15] The hospitals of the German universities are mostly owned and operated by the state, but in some instances, as at Hamburg and Cologne, they are largely municipal. The members of the professorial staff of these hospitals are state officers, and are largely withdrawn from contact with the medical profession. In the case of the younger members of the medical staff, their situation is made more difficult by the provision that no physician with a salary

INSURANCE IN CONTINENTAL EUROPE

of over 500 marks per month may engage in insurance practice.[16] This has required the withdrawal of some of the younger men from hospital work. Some 65 per cent of the patients in these hospitals are paid for out of the Insurance Funds, at the rate of 6.80 marks a day; the actual per capita cost is about 11 marks per day.[17] This provision for the care of patients sent in by the Funds, at rates significantly below the actual cost, is an arrangement common to continental hospital systems. It is, of course, a method of throwing part of the cost of hospital care onto taxation and, to that extent, relieves the Funds.

THE PHYSICIANS

In 1928 there were 48,507 physicians.[18] Of these, about 25 per cent were classified as specialists.[19] The nature of their practice has been mainly determined, of late years, by the national system of sickness insurance. Due to the increase of hospitals and hospital care, and the existence of large systems of school medical inspection, and child welfare, tuberculosis, maternity, and venereal disease supervision, practice has tended to become more and more official. It is said that only about 5 per cent of the physicians obtain their income wholly from private practice; 15 per cent are full-time government officials; while the remaining 80 per cent draw their income largely, or entirely, from the Insurance Funds.[20]

On the whole, the medical profession in Germany is well organized. There are many organizations, some of the Reich, some of the State, and some of the city—as in the case of Berlin—so that there is considerable overlapping. Some of the most important of the medical organizations have practically their whole reason for being in the necessity for organizations with which to combat the growing power of the *Krankenkassen*.

On the question of professional income, it is very difficult to obtain an unprejudiced opinion. Many or most of the statements on the subject are biased in one or the other direction. Furthermore, income varies a great deal in different sections of the country. Simons and Sinai[21] ("The Way of Health Insurance") quote an expert of the International Labor Office—who had compared the incomes in Germany with the incomes as found by the Committee on the Cost of Medical Care in Detroit—to the effect that incomes in the two countries were about the same. Dr. René Sand, of the League of Red Cross Societies, expresses the opinion that the average income of German physicians is about 11,000 marks—equal to $2,680. This computation would appear to agree with the previous citation, to the effect that average incomes in the two countries were not far from the same, when everything was taken into consideration.

The methods of payment under compulsory health insurance are of considerable variety. Thus there are six methods, any of which may be followed in any particular case: [22] (1) payment by attendance; (2) a capitation fee per insured person (similar to the "panel" system in England); (3) the same as (2), except that the capitation payments are paid into a fund from which the physicians are paid according to their actual attendance; (4) payment per case of sickness; (5) payment by fixed salaries; (6) full-time salary. Of these various methods, some are utilized by one organization, some by another. They also vary in different parts of the country.

RELATION OF THE PHYSICIANS TO THE KRANKENKASSEN

This relation can only be properly described as a more or less continuous guerilla warfare. At the outset, in Germany, as in most other countries, the medical profession was unprepared and unorganized, so that its case could not even be clearly stated. Since that time, the profession has been organized in various ways and has been better able to make its demands effective. It will be noted that the physicians in Germany deal directly with the *Krankenkassen,* and not, as in Great Britain, with the government. Obviously the interests of the two parties are widely divergent. The *Krankenkassen* desire to keep down the cost of medical care, while the physicians are attempting to see that a fee scale is maintained commensurate with the dignity of the profession. With the more or less steady increase in the amount of insurance practice, and with the gradual inclusion of more and more persons under this system, the power in the hands of the *Krankenkassen* has become very great.

Also, the War, with its aftermath of increasing social insurance, undoubtedly has made the working out of this program more difficult than would have been the case under normal conditions. It is conceivable that, in a long era of peace, the difficulties inherent in the organization might have been successfully overcome. However, under the conditions which have actually existed, no satisfactory adjustment has been attained. With the growth in the size and power of the *Krankenkassen* has gone a large increase in their overhead and their personnel. The latter has been increased, due to the alleged necessity of keeping careful track of the very complicated systems of payment, and of enabling the societies to decide whether or not the employed physicians were working in the interests of the society. As a result of various quarrels with the medical profession, the *Krankenkassen* have built hospitals, organized and built clinics for ambulatory patients, and employed full-time physicians to operate them. These clinics have now been largely discontinued as the result of pressure brought upon the government, but they constitute a continual threat of return to full-time paid service.

As already suggested, a large part of the difficulty arises as the result of the dual provision for medical care and sickness benefit. If the physician desires to keep upon his list the largest number of patients and consequently draw the largest income, it will obviously be in his interest to take a rather complaisant view of the duration of disability, and here, as under other systems, the tendency of disability claims to grow during periods of unemployment is very striking. The interest of the *Krankenkassen* is, obviously, to keep the periods of disability as short as possible, and physicians are under constant pressure to terminate the disability even though such termination, in their judgment, may be doubtfully in the interests of the patient. In the same way, a physician with a large insurance practice is tempted to do slipshod work and to indulge in overprescribing. This tendency is closely watched by the insurance societies, which have on their pay rolls a considerable number of full-time physicians whose business it is to watch the work of the insurance physicians. If the societies and the physicians were in full agreement, such oversight might be conducted in a perfectly satisfactory and amicable way, but where, as has commonly been the case in Germany, the physicians and the societies are at loggerheads, the physicians attached to the societies take on somewhat the character of spies.

There is apparently agreement among students of the situation that, under this system, the amount and duration of sickness have increased. This increase may be explained, of course, in two ways. The opponents of compulsory insurance commonly pointed to the increase in claims for very slight illness, and in the proportion of cases actual malingering. On the other hand, supporters of the system hold that, under the previous system, there was a very large group of sick people requiring medical service which they did not receive. As is so often the case, it is probable that both of these arguments contain a considerable element of truth. There is considerable evidence to show that under the system now operating in Germany the patients are definitely better off than before insurance was put into practice. There is ample evidence that the very large amount of neglect, prevalent in an earlier day, has now ceased and that, on the whole, the German people receive a much larger amount of satisfactory care. Particularly is this true in the case of the provision for hospital and specialist service, as well as in the provision for the care of tuberculosis. It cannot, I think, be denied that one result of the German system has been to increase, to a very desirable extent, the machinery—hospitals, sanatoria, and polyclinics—for the care of the sick.

When one comes to consider the effect of the system upon the physicians, the outlook is not so favorable. It is certainly true that the private practice of medicine has steadily diminished under this system and, at the present time, approaches the vanishing point. In this way, the freedom of action of the physician has become very much curtailed, and he constantly finds himself in conflict with a business organization whose chief concern may well appear to be the keeping down of expenses. The conscientious physician, who tries to apportion his time in relation to the actual needs of his patient, is likely to find himself at a disadvantage, as compared with his colleague who is content to spend the minimum time on the maximum number of patients. Hasty and ill-considered diagnosis, or, in fact, no diagnosis at all, may in this way become to the financial advantage of the physician. This difficulty, of course, is not peculiar to the system, since it exists in other countries where private practice is still the chief method. It is not clear that any system will prevent careless work by physicians whose interest is predominantly financial. A very full discussion of the shortcomings of the system from the point of view of the physicians has been made by Dr. Liek of Danzig.[23] A somewhat different view will be obtained from the publication of Drs. Goldmann and Grotjahn.[24] The situation suggests that it has become at once so complicated and, at least from the medical point of view, so unsatisfactory, that the new government of Germany may well be forced to a reorganization of the whole program.

XI

HEALTH INSURANCE IN THE BRITISH ISLES

The arrangements for medical care in the British Isles will be treated somewhat more fully than those in other countries, particularly as regards voluntary and compulsory health insurance, since its problems are more akin to our own. The basic similarity of language and common law makes their methods of dealing with the problems more likely to be suggestive and of interest for us.

England, Wales, and Northern Ireland

At the outset it is important to appreciate the British system of government, and the important respects in which it differs from that of the United States. It is essentially a democratic form of government, based upon representatives elected by adult suffrage. The legislative department of government is vested in the House of Commons, elected at a general election every four or five years, and the House of Lords, membership in which is hereditary. The House of Commons is much the more powerful body, because it is widely representative. Britain has a party government centered around the Prime Minister, who is the leader of the party in power. The work of the government is apportioned among a cabinet selected by the Prime Minister, the members of which have seats in Parliament. Any member is subject to interrogation in Parliament, a method which keeps the public very satisfactorily informed of the policies of the party in power. The Prime Minister and his Government remain in power only so long as they can command a majority in the House of Commons. If this majority fails them on a Government measure of any importance, the Government falls and is replaced through appointment, by the King, of the leader of the party to which power has apparently fallen. The fall of a Government and its replacement by another is ordinarily followed, after a reasonable period, by a general election. This method assures a quick response to changes of public opinion. On the whole the governments of Great

Britain are relatively stable as compared with those of many Continental countries.

Authority may be either central, derived from acts of Parliament, or local operated by local units. The relation of the central to the local government is carried on through what is known as the Civil Service. This is a system of permanent pensionable officers appointed by the Parliamentary Minister. They do not change with the fall of a Government, and, to this extent, are non-political officers. Through their permanency of tenure and the arrangement for pension, they form a most important body of administrators. The result is that these positions are held by men of great ability, and, as time goes on, of great experience. It will be noted that in this respect their position is entirely different from that of the various undersecretaries and assistant secretaries in our national government, who of necessity change with the party in power and, thus, periodically uproot the management of the country. This difference is important, since through our system it is relatively difficult to obtain men of commanding ability for such positions, and even though the services of such men be obtained, their tenure of office is rarely more than eight years, often not more than four. This principle of the Civil Service extends widely throughout the British System of Government, and as it is applied to officials high in administrative positions, differs radically from what is referred to as the Civil Service in this country. With us the Civil Service applies only to a relatively large group of minor officials.

The only government ministry with which we need here be much concerned is the Ministry of Health, which has the general oversight of public health, of destitution, of sickness insurance, and of the board of midwives.

Local government.—The Public Health Act of 1872 divided the country into urban and rural sanitary districts. The larger urban units were named boroughs. These units are governed by representatives elected by the direct votes of the ratepayers of each district. In 1888 county councils were created for the governing of the larger areas, and at the same time the largest boroughs were renamed county boroughs. The members of the county councils, county borough councils, the borough councils, and the urban and rural district councils, are elected for a definite period, usually for three years. One-third retire each year, so as to obtain continuity.

The local public health powers are exercised through the county borough councils, of which there are 82, and the county councils, which include the smaller units, to the number of 62.

Expenses of government.—There are two sources of government fund: taxes, which are levied by the central government, and rates, which are levied by the local government. The rates, a tax on land and buildings, are the only levy which the local authorities can exact. Recently, agricultural land has been exempt from this taxation, and there are some other special partial exemptions. This limitation of the local power of taxation might prove a serious handicap were it not for the system of government grants-in-aid, which may be given to local political areas for a great variety of purposes. It is important to note that considerable grants-in-aid are given for the care and management of tuberculosis, maternity and child welfare, and venereal disease.

ORGANIZATION OF THE MEDICAL PROFESSION

The General Medical Council was created by the General Medical Act of 1858, "An Act to regulate the qualifications of practitioners in medicine and surgery."[1] This act was modified, as concerns the composition of the General Medical Council, by the Act of 1886. As now constituted, the General Medical Council consists of one representative from each of the universities and colleges granting diplomas and degrees, five representatives of the central government, and three representatives of the medical practitioners, elected by vote of the practitioners of the United Kingdom. This council has wide supervisory powers over medical education. It is required to set up a Register of qualified practitioners in the United Kingdom and the British Empire. Only those physicians whose names are on the Register have the legal right to collect fees by legal process, if that be necessary. It will be noted that under this arrangement there is no prohibition of practice by any person not on the Register. On the other hand, such a person cannot hold any medical appointment, and cannot sign any certificate required by act of Parliament. These limitations place them under a serious handicap. As they cannot hold any appointment under the government, they are automatically barred from appointment under the insurance acts. It should be noticed that this system is in important contrast with the system of licensure adopted in this country. The General Medical Council is also concerned with questions of discipline, and charges brought against physicians on the Register. They sit as a trial board, hearing evidence and imposing penalties, which may vary from warning to removal from the Register.

The British Medical Association.—The British Medical Association is a voluntary organization having no statutory powers. In 1929 there were 34,979 members, of whom 22,080 were in England, Scotland, and Wales, and 1,020, in Ireland. (The balance of the membership is widely scattered throughout the Empire.) This number represented about 60 per cent of the physicians in Great Britain and Ireland, at that time. It represented a somewhat larger percentage of the general practitioners. The British Medical Association has played an outstanding part in the development of compulsory health insurance in Great Britain. When the Insurance Bill was brought forward in Parliament in 1911 the Association voiced its opposition and objections. The Bill was, however, passed in spite of this opposition. Since that time the coöperation between the British Medical Association and the Ministry of Health has been most excellent. Any careful reading of the discussions between these two bodies will show that, on both sides, there have been good temper, wisdom, and continuous consideration of public policy. Reference to the relations of these two bodies will be made later, since the history of their development has valuable lessons for other countries, in regard to the relationship between government and medical practice.

Medical Officers of Health.—These officers hold positions similar to those which in this country would be occupied by public health officers. However, their status and relations differ in important respects. In Great Britain they may be appointees either of the central (Ministry of Health) or the local health authorities. In the country areas, the county boroughs, and the large boroughs, they are full-time medical officers removable only for cause—such as gross misconduct—and are entitled to a pension. In the smaller towns, the medical officers of health are commonly part-time officers, often being general practitioners, who do the work in conjunction with their practice. In these smaller towns, they are often responsible to the medical officers of health in the county areas. This is in important contrast to the position of most public health officers in this country, whose appointments are tenuous to a degree, and depend upon local shifts of political power, so that their security is chiefly characterized by its absence. As was noted above in regard to the Civil Service, the British system of security of tenure makes these positions much to be desired, and they do in fact command the services of able people.

The relation of the practicing physicians to the medical officers of health is similar to that which obtains in this country with the public health officers. To them, the physicians report births, deaths, and infectious disease. They are also entitled to secure from the medical officers of health assistance in the diagnosis of doubtful cases of infectious disease, to obtain the officially provided assistance in bacteriologic tests, X ray examinations, and consultation with medical officers of official clinics.

HOSPITALS

The hospital system of Great Britain is of particular interest because in many ways its growth has been similar, though with important differences, to the development of hospitals in this country.

The voluntary hospital.—This is the term generally applied to the many hospitals in Great Britain founded and maintained by the gifts of charitably inclined persons. (In this country they are commonly referred to as charity hospitals.) Their origin dates back to the Middle Ages, when they often sprang up from ecclesiastical foundations. They represent in Great Britain, as in this country, the doctrine of *noblesse oblige*, under which the more opulent members of the community feel required to contribute to the medical care of those less fortunately situated.

In 1924, there were some 847 voluntary hospitals in England and Wales, with some 50,460 beds—which is, roughly speaking, 1.3 beds per 1,000 of the population. These voluntary hospitals have an enormous dispensary service, corresponding to the great out-patient departments of the charity hospitals in this country. In the London

Area, for instance, there were, according to a recent report, 136 such hospitals, with an in-patient rate of 43.9 per 1,000, and a bed rate of 3.17 per 1,000. In 1926, the new out-patients visiting these hospitals were 355 per 1,000. The situation of these voluntary hospitals as regards financial support has become increasingly difficult since the War. Generally speaking, up to that time, the prosperity of Great Britain was such that the support of these institutions was relatively secure. But due to the heavy, increasing income and inheritance taxes, it is obvious that the source of supply is gradually drying up, and that in Great Britain, as in this country, hospital provision will have to fall increasingly upon the public. Of recent years, there has developed a tendency on the part of these hospitals to collect part of the cost from patients, a system which until relatively recent times was not practiced. As originally founded, these hospitals were intended for the indigent, and were so used. With the shrinking of the sources of their support, it has become increasingly necessary to depend upon charges to patients—although even as yet these charges defray but a small proportion of the cost. From a recent report it would appear that something like 24 per cent of the income of the voluntary hospitals was thus obtained; some 28 per cent of their income was from voluntary gifts; some 18 per cent, from investments; and some 10 per cent, from legacies. Of late years, the balance of their income has been derived from central funds and from an increasing development of voluntary hospital insurance, under which people in moderate circumstances assure themselves hospital accommodations in case of severe illness. This insurance is offered to people with incomes varying from £4 a week, in the case of single persons, to £6 a week for persons with families. The contributions are ordinarily about 3d. a week (about 6 cents), or about 12s. a year. This development is due, at least partly, to the fact that the National Insurance Act makes no provision for hospital care, and, except in the case of the necessitous, such hospital care has to be arranged for in other ways.

Official hospitals.—This group includes all hospitals supported by government. In 1928, the bed capacity was roughly as follows: isolation and port sanitary hospitals, 38,200; tuberculosis hospitals and convalescent homes, 22,655; hospitals for mental disease, 139,122;

county council hospitals, 120,235—making a grand total of 320,212. The County Council Hospitals are those which, prior to 1930, were known as Poor Law Hospitals, and corresponded roughly to the city and county hospitals of this country.

OFFICIAL MEDICAL ASSISTANCE FOR THE NECESSITOUS

A well-developed system built up over many years exists for the care of people whose immediate condition requires medical attention for which they cannot afford to pay, but who may not necessarily be permanently indigent. The distinction may be an important one. This care is under the supervision of the Public Assistance Committees of the Counties and County Boroughs, and the Public Health Committees of the County Councils. The domiciliary care is carried out by, or under the supervision of, the District Medical Officer, who is a salaried official with security of tenure, who cannot be dismissed without the approval of the Ministry of Health, and who is entitled to a pension. From a recent report it appears that there are some 3,400 such officers in England and Wales. These physicians may or may not be full-time. Many of the District Medical Officers are general practitioners who hold the position in addition to their private practice. In the more thickly settled communities these officers tend more frequently to become full-time salaried people. Where hospital care or specialized service is required, the District Medical Officer makes the necessary arrangements with the public assistance hospitals. These hospitals have a full-time medical officer in charge, and, as a rule, a full-time medical staff sufficient to carry on the work. Many of them also have a visiting and consulting staff, which may or may not be paid an honorarium. By this arrangement there has been set up the machinery necessary to provide pretty satisfactory care for necessitous patients not included under the National Insurance Act, and through the development of hospitals for tuberculosis, and provision for mental and venereal disease, the setup is relatively complete and satisfactory.

INSURANCE MEDICAL SERVICE

In considering the conditions which led to the establishment of the British Insurance Medical Service it is important to realize the condition of the medical service at an earlier day. A great deal of the unfavorable comment, which has been made in the United States concerning the British Compulsory Insurance System, has overlooked the conditions which existed in Great Britain prior to the Act of 1911. Few Americans realize the congested conditions and unsatisfactory housing situation in the large industrial cities in the England of that day. Still fewer realize the extent to which the medical care through the agency of the old Friendly Societies had been developed. As early as 1815, these Friendly Societies had a membership of 925,439. They were friendly societies, in the most literal sense of the word, in that the members and management of these societies felt a very deep personal interest in the members. There was a strong tendency on the part of the members to avoid "going on the society" except for very real conditions of illness. By 1904 the membership of these societies had risen to 5,700,000—which is more than one-third of the number of people now entitled to benefit under the Insurance Act. The medical care given by these societies was under a system of contract with physicians, these contracts paying from 3*s.* to 4*s.* (75 cents to $1.00) per member per year. For this sum, the contract doctor gave medical care, plus necessary medicines. Though the compensation was not large, there was sharp competition among the physicians for this work, particularly in the large industrial cities, and by an undesirable system of bidding against each other they tended to lower their own compensation. The system, though undoubtedly better than nothing, was unsatisfactory for two reasons: In the first place, the membership of these societies tended to include chiefly the careful and provident people, whereas the careless and improvident were likely to be either wholly without medical service, or dependent upon the medical service provided by the poor law authorities. In the second place, on account of the competition among physicians for this work, their compensation was likely to be small; their number of patients, large; and the temptation to do slipshod work, great. In most respects, the service thus given did not differ importantly from that which has been contributed in other countries on similar systems and which has nowhere proved satisfactory in the long run.

The investigation which led to the establishment of the Insurance

Medical Service came about as the result of the Report of the Royal Commission on the Poor Laws in 1909. This was intended to be a study of the problems of indigence rather than the problems of health. This will tend to explain some of the weaknesses of the law and, to some extent, the incompleteness of the service. It has been almost universally true that the approach by the public to the problems of the health of people in the lower income-brackets has been from the side of indigence rather than from the side of improvements in the public health. It is, of course, evident that the problems of indigence involving poor housing and sanitary conditions are intimately related to those of health. On the other hand, where the approach is from the side of poverty, important public health aspects are likely to be overlooked, because the committees, or commissions, are insufficiently equipped with experts in this field. This will also tend to explain the failure, which has been almost universal, to consult the medical profession sufficiently early and sufficiently widely, for the purpose of giving to the undertaking a sound and broad base, from the point of view of the public health. As a rule, the medical profession, if called in at all, has been called in late in the inquiry and, unfortunately, has frequently been inadequately prepared to answer the questions put to them. Thus, legislation of an inadequate type has often resulted.

The National Insurance Act.—This Act which was the outcome of the Report of the Royal Commission on the Poor Laws, two years earlier, was passed in 1911 under the unfavorable conditions suggested above. It was hastily prepared under the, then, Chancellor of the Exchequer, Mr. Lloyd George. It obtained inadequate discussion and was violently opposed, at the outset, by the British Medical Association, which had not been given an adequate opportunity to consult on the terms of the Act. Since its original passage, many changes have been made as the result of conference between the representatives of the British Medical Association and the Ministry of Health. A careful reading of the discussions which have taken place between the representatives of the British Medical Association and Sir George Newman, Undersecretary to the Ministry of Health, and principal medical officer of the Ministry of Health, will show the very great advantages which can accrue from such conferences.

In this case they have been conducted on a very high plane and have shown clear recognition, on both sides, of the importance of considering the benefit to accrue to the people at large—not losing sight of the importance of maintaining the position and dignity of the profession.

Scope of the Act.—The Act covers employed persons over sixteen years of age with an income below £250 (about $1,250). At first, it included only industrial employees, but has since been modified to include small tradespeople, more or less independent groups involved in the fishing trades, and domestic servants. It thus covers about fifteen million employed persons—about one-third of the population and which, it will be remembered, is less than three times the number of people previously included in the contract work provided by the Friendly Societies. The weekly payments under the Act are 1*s.* 6*d.* for men (about 36 cents) and 1*s.* 1*d.* (about 26 cents) for women. Of this, one-half is contributed by the employer and one-half by the employee. The insurance thus provided covers the Medical Benefit, the Widows' and Orphans' Benefit, and the Old-Age Pension, which accrues to employed persons reaching the age of sixty-five after which their contributions cease.

Management of the Insurance Act.—The management of the Insurance Act is in the hands of three authorities: the Ministry of Health, the Insurance Committees, and the Approved Societies.

THE APPROVED SOCIETIES

At their inception, the approved societies consisted of the old Friendly Societies and the societies built up by trade unions. To these were added Industrial Insurance Societies, which were in fact insurance companies, doing a life insurance business, who added industrial insurance to their other work. This was, on the whole, objectionable, since they brought into the group of societies a purely commercial atmosphere. It was provided under the Act that these societies should be on a nonprofit-making basis, and to this requirement the life insurance companies subscribed, conducting a separate department for the industrial insurance work which was valuable to them chiefly because it brought their agents in contact with a very large number of people, many of whom, as in the case of the family of the insured, were not covered by the Act. A recent return shows that 46.5 per cent of the Approved Societies are Friendly Societies, with or without branches throughout the United Kingdom, 24.8 per cent are Industrial Insurance Societies, and about 10.7 per cent are made up of Trade Unions and Employers' Provident Funds. There are in all over 1,000 Approved Societies, the membership of which may vary from as few as 50 to over two million. The business of these societies is to collect and pay out the monetary benefits accruing under the Act. The large societies in England, as is the case in Germany, wield very considerable political power. Undoubtedly, it would have been better if the Insurance Act had been organized directly under the Ministry of Health without the intervention of these societies. Such an arrangement, however, was probably impossible since the Act, as initiated by Mr. Lloyd George, had a very considerable political slant to it, and the political power already possessed by the Friendly Societies was essential to insure its passage. Though the matter will be more fully discussed later, it is proper to point out at this time that the political phases of the various compulsory insurance arrangements in Europe have been important handicaps to the most effective methods of organization. Though the British Medical Association was ill prepared to present its case effectively at the time the Act was under consideration, it still succeeded in forcing upon the government an arrangement by which the physicians dealt directly with the Ministry of Health, and not, as under the German arrangement, with the Approved Societies. This is undoubtedly one reason why the British Insurance Act has worked better than the German.

THE LOCAL INSURANCE COMMITTEES

These were provided for under the Act, one for each county and county borough. There are at the present time 146 in England and Wales, and 45 in Scotland. The membership of these committees, as provided for in the Act, required that three-fifths of the members be elected by the Approved Societies, one-fifth by the County Council, two medical members elected by the medical profession, one medical member appointed by the Council, several members appointed by the Ministry of Health, including two women. It was the original intention of the Act that the medical profession should deal with this committee, but the British Medical Association insisted, from the start, that it must deal directly with the Ministry of Health. Thus, a part of the powers originally intended for these committees has not been exercised. As far as professional questions are concerned, the Ministry of Health acts as the intermediary between the insurance committee and the physicians. The duties of the Local Insurance Committee are chiefly three: (1) to prepare and publish a list of physicians and druggists registered on the panel, (2) to prepare for publication a list of the patients on each physician's panel, (3) the pricing of prescriptions for which the druggists are paid under the Act.

In each area there is a Local Medical Committee which is made up of representatives of the physicians. The Local Insurance Committee must consult this committee on all professional questions. The local Medical Committee is purely advisory. Also, in each area, there is a subcommittee of the Local Insurance Committee, the business of which is to hear complaints arising in regard to the medical management of the Act. This subcommittee is composed of an equal number of representatives of the societies and of the physicians. If this committee is unable to come to a satisfactory agreement, the matter is referred for adjudication to the Ministry of Health, which hears the question with the advice of an advisory committee including insurance physicians. That there are relatively few complaints arising under this Act is shown by the fact that in 1928 there were only 299 such cases in England and Wales; of those, only 42 cases were referred to the Ministry of Health. All of the hearings on complaints are private. In practice, only the cases in which some disciplinary action against a physician is contemplated are referred to the Ministry of Health.

THE MINISTRY OF HEALTH

The Ministry of Health is headed by a cabinet minister belonging to the party in power. In practice, the business of the Minister of Health is to interpret to Parliament the problems of his department, including the administration of the Insurance Act. The real business of the department is carried on by the permanent Civil Service officers of the department headed by the Undersecretary of the Ministry of Health and the principal medical officer of the Ministry. This position has for many years been held by Sir George Newman, a distinguished authority on public health problems and, also, on the problems of medical education. To him has fallen, very largely, the adjudication of the problems arising under this hastily passed Act, and to him, in no small measure, belongs the credit for the satisfactory workings of the Act at the present time. It is, of course, not to be expected that the Ministry of Health will always be so fortunate as to have so able a person in this position, but his administration gives ample evidence of the value of these permanent undersecretaries and their essential importance in the smooth working of any problem so complicated as health insurance.

BENEFITS UNDER THE INSURANCE ACT

The payments made by the insured entitle him to benefits of two kinds: (1) the money benefits, which consist of a sickness allowance, a disablement allowance, a maternity benefit, and an old-age pension; (2) medical benefits. It is important to distinguish between these two types of benefit since their management by the same machinery and using the same physicians has given rise to some of the most knotty problems in administration.

The sickness benefits.—This benefit is 15s. ($3.75) a week for men and 12s. ($3.00) a week for women, payment beginning upon the fourth day and continuing up to twenty-six weeks. The disablement benefit is an allowance of 7s. 6d. ($1.87) a week, payable after the sickness allowance has lapsed. This may be continued for an indefinite period. The maternity benefit consists in a payment of £2 ($10.00) to an insured woman, or to the wife of an insured man. There is an additional payment of £2 ($10.00) to a married employed woman. The old-age benefit, as above noted, is payable after the age of sixty-five.

The medical benefit.—The medical benefit consists in the provision of medical care of such type and grade as can be furnished by the general practitioner, and does not involve the application of special skill of a kind not reasonably to be expected of the general practitioner. It provides for domiciliary visits, and care at the physician's office. The local panel of physicians is composed of all physicians on the Register who desire to do panel practice. There are about 38,000 practitioners on the Medical Register. In England and Wales there are about 18,000 general practitioners, and 15,276 of these were, according to a recent report, doing some panel practice.

Scope of medical service.—As above pointed out, the service provided is that which can be given by the general practitioner. The patients have complete freedom of choice among the physicians, and a physician may refuse to accept a patient on his panel. The number of patients who may be accepted by a given physician is limited to 2,500, though an additional 1,500 may be taken on the panel if the physician employs a full-time paid assistant. A patient may transfer from the panel of one physician to another after giving fourteen days' notice of his intention. It will be seen that this, though a necessary and desirable provision, creates a large amount of bookkeeping for the Insurance Committee which is required to post a correct list of the patients on the panels of the various physicians. The ordinary rules of medical practice obtain in regard to a physician who desires to discontinue his treatment of a patient. He may do so, after having assured himself that the patient has been accepted on the panel of another physician and after proper conference with his colleague. In the unusual case of a physician desiring to disengage himself from a patient, and being unable to place him upon the panel of another physician, the matter is referred to the Local Insurance Committee, which will make compulsory allocation. The medical benefit is quite incomplete in that it makes no provision for hospital care, or for consultation or care by specialists. Panel physicians sometimes offer to provide, on the ordinary basis of private practice, services not furnished under the Act. This they may do, but they are required to notify the Insurance Committee within two days after they have done so. The Insurance Committee is then at liberty to decide that these services should have been included under the scope of the Act, in which case the physician can make no extra charge for his services. The panel physicians do not furnish obstetrical care, though a monetary benefit is paid to the insured, or the wife of the insured, for such service.

Remuneration.—The remuneration of practitioners under the Insurance Act is on a capitation basis, that is to say, there is a fixed sum paid for each person on the physician's panel. This payment was originally fixed at 7s. 6d. ($1.87) per year per insured person. In 1924 it was raised to 9s. ($2.25). As there is a separate provision for medicines and drugs under the Act, these are not furnished by the physician, and he is certain of retaining the full sum paid by the government. The element of bad debts which is always a considerable item in the overhead of the physician is in this way entirely avoided. In 1928, the average income of the panel physicians was £447 (about $2,235.00). This sum compares favorably with the average income of general practitioners in the United States. All the testimony goes to show that the income of the practitioner doing panel work has been substantially increased by the Act. There is no prohibition against the panel physicians doing any amount of private practice, provided, of course, that this practice is not upon patients within the scope of the Insurance Act. It thus arises that physicians with large panels earn a very satisfactory income from this practice alone, while physicians with smaller panels, often because they do not desire to do a large amount of this type of practice, may still have a very satisfactory income from private practice.

TOTAL EXPENSE OF MEDICAL CARE

In 1928 there were about 15,276 doctors and 9,000 chemists' shops furnishing medical care under the Act. At the same time there were about 13,900,000 persons on the panels. The total payments to panel physicians were £6,831,300 (about $34,156,500.00). The chemists' shops received £2,241,780 (about $11,208,900.00). This represented a total expense per insured person of 9s. 10d. (about $2.45) for doctors' fees and 3s. 3d. (about $0.81) for medicines. In addition to these payments, country physicians received £300,000 (about $1,500,000.00) for extra mileage in visiting patients living a distance from their offices.

MEDICAL CERTIFICATION

Medical certification is certification for incapacity to work, and entitles the insured to payment for sickness disability, and for disability after the lapse of the sickness payment. The payment on account of this benefit in 1928 was some £20,000,000 ($100,000,-000.00). As already suggested, the certification for disability is one of the most troublesome parts of the situation created by the Compulsory Insurance Act. The difficulty arises because the physicians are acting, on the one hand, for their patients, and, on the other hand, for the insurance funds. During the period from 1921 to 1927 examination of the books of the insurance funds by the Government Actuary showed an increase in claims for sickness disability varying from 60 to 100 per cent. The increase in claims for men was 41 per cent, for unmarried women 60 per cent, and for married women 106 per cent. The increase was greater in the case of disability allowances; the figures were, respectively, 85 per cent, 100 per cent, and 159 per cent. Increases of this sort have been rather common under compulsory insurance in various countries. Undoubtedly part of the increase may be charged against the difficult economic conditions existing in Europe during this period, but part, at least, is evidence of a weakness of the system under which the physician is greatly tempted to take a somewhat lighthearted view of his responsibilities to the government. Some of the opinions held by those concerned with the administration of the Act may be gathered from the following quotation from the presidential address of Mr. F. Lewis, the president of the National Conference of Friendly Societies in September, 1930:

A large proportion of the insurance practitioners were giving to the insured persons treatment and attention that was commendable, but there were too many medical men whose treatment of insured persons was perfunctory and negligent, and some who were willing to do almost anything in order that they might secure a cheap popularity and a long panel list, even to the extent of assisting persons to obtain benefit to which they were not justly entitled.

Another such opinion may be taken from a recent issue of the *National Insurance Gazette:*

The average doctor takes the view that his patient engages him and that his sole duty is owed to that patient. That is the doctor's traditional attitude, and it was entirely correct in former times. It is only partly correct under the National Health Insurance system. The first part of the proposition is true, but the second part is not. The patient engages the doctor, but the whole body of insured persons pays the doctor's fees, and therefore a duty is owed to that body. The individual patient does not pay the doctor's bill. The whole body pays, and we put it to the doctors, as honest men, that a duty is owed to that body.

The Ministry of Health has on various occasions called the matter officially to the attention of panel physicians, pointing out their obligations to the government as well as to the patient.

REGIONAL MEDICAL OFFICERS

The Ministry of Health has a staff of fifty-nine full-time medical officers for England and Wales, distributed on a territorial basis. The most important duty of these officers is to examine patients referred to them either by the societies, or by the physicians, and concerning whom there is difference of opinion as to certification for disability. In this way, the regional medical officers act as medical referees. This appears to be a very desirable arrangement, because they are representatives neither of the societies nor of the physicians involved, and can come to opinions quite independent of the claims put forward on either side. In 1927, 312,580 such cases were referred to the regional medical officers, but of this number, only 176,751 appeared for examination, the remaining large fraction preferring to return to work rather than subject their cases to review. Of the number submitting to examination, 125,800 were found incapable of work, while the balance was refused further disability allowance.

An occasional source of irritation and disagreement in the adjudication of claims for disability allowance is the discrepancy between the amount allowed for disability and the amount allowed for unemployment insurance. The sickness disability is 15s. ($3.75) whereas the unemployment disability is 18s. ($4.50). Thus the payment is larger for unemployment than for disability.

In view of the rather frequent statements appearing in the medical press of this country, tending to indicate that the National Insurance Act of Great Britain is not working satisfactorily, it may be worthwhile to quote opinions from various sources which may be held to be competent witnesses. Thus, the report of the Royal Commission on National Health Insurance, in 1926, in the official evidence of the British Medical Association, states,

INSURANCE IN THE BRITISH ISLES

The evidence as to the incidence of sickness benefit does point to the fact that the scheme has almost certainly reduced national sickness, and we are quite sure that if the immense gain to national health includes immense gain to the comfort of the individual in knowing that he can have medical attention whenever he needs it, the gain is most marked.

The Commissioners expressed the following opinion: "We are satisfied that the scheme of National Health Insurance has fully justified itself and has, on the whole, been successful in operation."

In 1922 the British Medical Association, in stating its opinion that the benefit should be continued, said:

(a) Large numbers, indeed whole classes of persons are now receiving a real medical attention which they formerly did not receive at all.
(b) The number of practitioners in proportion to the population in densely populated areas has increased.
(c) The amount and character of the medical attention given is superior to that formerly given in the best of the old clubs, and immensely superior to that given in the great majority of the clubs which were far from the best.
(d) Illness is now coming under skilled observation and treatment at an earlier stage than was formerly the case.
(e) Speaking generally, the work of practitioners has been given a bias towards prevention which was formerly not so marked.
(f) Clinical records have been or are provided which may be made of great service in relation to medical research and public health.
(g) Coöperation among practitioners is being encouraged to an increasing degree.
(h) There is now a more marked recognition than formerly of the collective responsibility of the profession to the community in respect of all health matters.

Sir Arthur Newsholme, whose outstanding qualifications as a witness upon this question can hardly be doubted, says,

It can be accepted that for the majority of insured persons medical benefit as now administered has been a boon. For (a) every obstacle to early medical consultation and diagnosis has been removed; and (b) a serious source of anxiety—the expense of domiciliary medical attendance—no longer exists so far as concerns the wage-earner in each family.

These are important gains to set against the alleged inferior service under medical benefit. It is certain that some doctors—especially those with large panels—have their surgeries crowded during limited hours, and oft-times give a perfunctory interview, followed by the prescription of a bottle of medicine, not preceded by an adequate overhaul of the patient. In mitigation it may be said that persons of the same social class would, apart from insurance, receive similar treatment. This, of course, does not justify unsatisfactory contract work; and as the education of the insured improves, practitioners acting thus will lose in prestige and practice.

ADDITIONAL MEDICAL BENEFITS

Where the Approved Societies have surplus funds they are permitted to allow medical benefits not provided for in the Act. The societies are not authorized to provide treatment, but the panel physicians may indicate to their patients where and how these benefits may be obtained, and they will be paid for by the society, if it has a surplus, and if it approves of the benefit. The most common additional benefit is that of dental care, which was provided by over 6,000 funds, to an amount of £2,520,293 (about $12,601,465.00) in 1928. The next most common was the ophthalmic benefit, for which about one-sixth of that amount was contributed. Following this were allowances for hospitals, convalescent homes, surgical appliances, and nursing. It will be noted that there is here a definite departure from the plan under which medical benefits are provided, by physicians under direct arrangements with the government. These additional benefits are allowed by the societies if and when they have a surplus, and if and when they regard the request as appropriate. This more nearly approaches the relation between the physicians and the *Krankenkassen* in Germany, and has the effect of introducing the element of lay control and opinion into a problem which is in fact purely medical. Thus, an urgently needed benefit may be denied to an insured person whose society has no surplus; it may also be denied to an insured person whose society has a surplus, but whose officials doubt the wisdom of supplying it.

INCOMPLETENESS OF SERVICE

It is important to appreciate clearly that the service rendered under the Insurance Act is very far from a complete service, much less complete, in fact, than that given in Germany. It does not provide (1) hospital accommodations, (2) consultant service of specialists,

(3) laboratory examinations, or (4) nursing. This limitation of the service has been appreciated by all concerned. That it is recognized by the insured is shown by the quite extraordinary increase in voluntary insurance, particularly that which covers hospital care, in the period following the War. This rapid increase of insurance taken by persons covered by the Insurance Act is also an interesting commentary on the possibility of maintaining compulsory insurance and voluntary insurance, side by side. It may be taken as evidence that the insured persons have become convinced of the value of the insurance principle as applied to sickness.

By far the most important evidence of wide recognition of the incompleteness of the Insurance Act is the fact that in 1930 the British Medical Association put forward a plan for broad extension of the Act, to cover the above-mentioned factors not already included. If such an extension was undertaken, it would provide for a quite complete service at the income level of the present Act. That such a plan should be advised by the British Medical Association is evidence of the extent to which that group has become convinced of the soundness of the principle. It is probable that the expense involved, which would be very considerable, is the chief reason why such an extension has not been undertaken. It is not unlikely that extension of the Act along these lines may be expected when it becomes financially feasible.

OBSTETRICAL CARE

In surveying the medical service of Great Britain, it is important to note briefly the provisions for obstetrical care. For a long time, midwives have attended a large proportion of the confinements. For example, in 1869, 50 to 90 per cent of the total births were attended by midwives. In 1872 there was created a board for the supervision of midwives. The Midwives Act in 1902 created a Central Midwives Board for England and Wales. This provided for education and supervision of midwives, under rules which must be approved by the Ministry of Health. In 1927 there were 16,610 practicing midwives in England and Wales, and about 61 per cent of all the births in this area were attended by midwives. Under the regulations, midwives can only conduct uncomplicated confinements, and are required to call a registered physician should complications occur. These complications are carefully specified by the rules laid down under the Act. In case a midwife summons a physician to her assistance the local authority is required to pay that physician, in accordance with an approved scale of fees. Thus, it is seen that Great Britain has accepted the view that the midwife is an important part of the medical service, that, therefore, she should be properly trained, properly supervised, and that she should act in a proper relation to registered physicians. Lest it should be supposed that, as the result of the very large proportion of births tended by midwives, obstetrical care has suffered, it may be pointed out that the mortality statistics of patients confined by midwives compare very favorably with those of patients attended by physicians.

Scotland

The previous discussion was confined to the workings of the Insurance Act in England and Wales. In general, the machinery is the same in Scotland, but, since Scotland has a considerable measure of home rule, some of the details are different. For instance, in Scotland the Scottish Department of Health replaces, and has the powers exercised by, the Ministry of Health for England and Wales. In 1929 the population of Scotland was 4,842,544—more than one-fourth living in the city of Glasgow. In Scotland the National Insurance Act operates along similar lines to those in force in England, the important exception being what is known as the Highlands and Islands Medical Service. This developed in Scotland because of the large area with a sparse and scattered population, and the considerable number of islands lying off the coast. Medical service for these areas is essential, but the population would have difficulty in supporting a sufficient number of physicians. This service arose as the result of a survey by a government committee in 1912. In 1913 the Highlands and Islands Service was given a fund of £42,000 ($210,-000.00). This is used to make grants to practitioners to enable them to obtain a reasonable income, where this could not be supplied by the population. In some areas, which are spoken of as "single practice areas," the grant is made to the physician on the understanding that he will visit all individuals requiring medical care. For those unable to pay, a fee of 5s. ($1.25) is granted for the first visit, and

3s. 6d. ($0.87) for subsequent visits. Allowance is also made to the physicians for upkeep of motor cars, motorcycles, and motor boats. According to a recent report, there are 156 physicians working under this scheme of modified fees and, in addition, grants for mileage were made to twenty-four physicians. On the average the physicians receive about £260 ($1,300.00) annually from these grants. In 1927 the total payments from the fund—for medical service, nursing service, and various other special services—amounted to £69,921 ($349,605.00). The principle of subsidizing physicians in sparsely settled districts is of considerable interest. It appears to have assisted very much in solving the difficulty of maintaining medical service in outlying districts where, on the previous basis, it could not reasonably be expected that a physician would always, or even generally, be available. It is quite conceivable that such an arrangement might be used to advantage in various portions of the United States. A somewhat similar plan has been put into operation in portions of the Dominion of Canada.

XII

MEDICAL NEEDS IN THE UNITED STATES

In undertaking to discuss the medical needs of the country, it may as well be admitted at the outset that the word "needs" might easily be used in a variety of senses. It would be possible, for instance, to survey the situation with a view to ascertaining by how far the supply of medical service in this country fell short of an ideal standard. By the same token, an attempt might be made to prescribe the precise amount of medical service held to be requisite for satisfactory care of disease. Such inquiries might readily be of interest and importance, but they would deal, at best, with highly speculative situations, and would turn largely upon matters of opinion. It is perhaps true that *any* statement which may be made in this field will be based, to a considerable extent, on opinion—it is not humanly possible to be familiar with the great variety of medical problems which obviously exist in a country of this size. It may be proper, therefore, to admit at the outset that many of the conclusions which may be reached will be, at best, matters of opinion, and should be considered as such.

General Considerations

However, it seems to me beyond question that the problem must be discussed, not upon the plane of what medical service might theoretically be desirable, but what evidences of weakness can be presented, and of envisioning the conditions peculiar to this country which, for that reason, cannot be remedied by methods which may have proved satisfactory elsewhere. The best consideration which I have been able to give to the subject has brought me definitely to the conclusion that the interests of the country, as regards improvement of its medical service, must be studied in the light of local conditions, and that the conclusions ultimately reached probably will be considerably at variance with what might be judged to be necessary or desirable elsewhere. I cannot convince myself that the conditions in this country can be satisfactorily met by transplanting plans which are, at least apparently, satisfactory in other countries. In the first place, the area is larger than that of any other country which has squarely faced its medical problems for any considerable period. There are regions of pretty dense population, though few, which correspond closely with many of the European countries. As against these, there are vast areas of scattered population for which it seems essential to make plans, at least hopefully, in the direction of more complete service, and which, as far as I am aware, have no close parallel elsewhere.

Quite apart from questions of population density and geography are the general questions of the average level of education. Broadly speaking, the level of education in this country is high as compared with any other countries with anything like the same area. The extent to which newspapers and magazines are circulated and read is on the whole very great, and, finally, a method of circulating information very widely has of late years developed by means of the radio. I believe it to be a safe assertion that it is on the whole more possible in this country to obtain wide diffusion of information—one may hesitate to say knowledge—than anywhere else. This fact must importantly influence any plans which may be put forward for supplying medical service. The desirable diffusion of information is to some extent counterbalanced by the large amount of misinformation which is also received through the same sources. The patent medicine and the quack have flourished in this country, in part at least, because of the advertising which they have obtained through the newspapers.

It will be safe to assume that a handsome proportion of the population, at any given time, will be fairly well informed as to possible methods of dealing with disease. The medical profession in this country will, on the whole, have to keep itself more closely in step with modern progress than has been the case elsewhere. Furthermore, I have the impression that the average adult in this country is more interested in science, is more likely to have some—though probably very incomplete—knowledge of at least the jargon of science, and is more likely to demand that scientific discovery be made available in the treatment of disease, than anywhere else in the world. If this impression be correct, it will require of those who propose to improve medical service that this state of mind be taken fairly into account. Some study of the problems in Europe leads me to the opinion that a grade of medical service which is apparently entirely satisfactory, and probably fairly meets the demand in various of those countries, would fall short of the demand here, and would prove unsatisfactory.

It does not appear to me to be accidental that the subdivision of the fields of medicine and the development of specialization have on the whole gone considerably further in this country than abroad. It is not intended to suggest that the United States has any monopoly of the great experts in any field, for such is not the case, but I believe it to be true, that in relation to the total number of physicians, there is a larger proportion who have limited their field and are qualified to be regarded as specialists.

This may be a consequence of the common observation that, as a people, we are mechanically minded, and have shown more than average aptitude in those things which can be dealt with in mechanical ways and which require manual dexterity. Now, of course, there are many special fields of medicine which cannot be mastered by mechanical mindedness, and which do require profound knowledge and careful thinking. Opposed to this, however, is a considerable group, particularly of the so-called surgical specialties, in which unusual technical skill and mechanical ability are very considerably at a premium.

It seems fair, therefore, to suggest that, in any even hasty survey of the medical needs of this country, they must be approached largely on the basis of conditions as they actually exist, that we must concern ourselves with supplying, not a grade of medical service which has apparently been satisfactory elsewhere, but try to visualize the types of practice and the provisions of service which are most nearly consonant with the actual demand. Perhaps a somewhat different reading of the same text may account for the fact that there is apparently no other country in the world which has been so bedeviled with irregular practitioners, and in which such a large proportion of the funds expended for alleged medical purposes are spent upon patent medicines. One can hardly avoid the conclusion that this development has been due to the extent to which the American people read advertisements, to a certain childlike faith in the honesty of newspaper advertising, and to a great deal of publicity, which though in fact advertising does not obviously appear as such. Thus, we are forced to the conclusion, which must always be reluctantly reached by any student of economic problems, that many of the most difficult questions in the development of satisfactory health service will have to be worked out in this country largely on the basis of its own experience, drawing relatively little from the experience of others, and consequently depending somewhat for its ultimate success on trial and error. Having made these perhaps damaging admissions, an attempt will here be made to indicate certain weaknesses of our present organization.

Community Health

Community health may be distinguished from individual health as being that aspect of health service which deals with groups rather than with individuals and which must be overseen by those medical organizations which we speak of as the public health services. Great advance has been made in this country, in the last thirty years, in the direction of putting at the disposal of the community, medical men with at least some special training in the field of public health who can supervise those portions of the field which must be dealt with in bulk, rather than through individual service. But, though we have come a considerable distance along the road, it is probably true that we are still less well equipped than are many of the Old World countries. Certain it is that, though we have under our noses the evidence of the tremendous value of public health service in the diminution of contagious disease, as a people we are still very far from recognizing the value of this part of medical service. It would seem elementary that a physician who has obtained the necessary training to qualify him as an expert in the field of public health should have a reasonable opportunity of devoting his life to this special service, but this has been very much less possible than it should have been, probably, on account of our form of government. Obviously, a health officer must be employed by a political subdivision, which may vary from the national government to the smallest political unit. It would appear equally obvious that if we are to expect good service, we must offer to these people considerable security of tenure. In many European countries such officers are appointed by political units of any size, after careful selection, and are given life appointments, and pensions. In this way, if the selection of such officers is wisely carried out and if a good educational background is insisted upon, excellent service may be expected.

The habit of this country, however, has been very different. Commonly enough, the health officers of any unit below that of the United States Public Health Service are purely political employees, beholden to the party or group temporarily in power, and having no security beyond that which they may be able to obtain by trimming their sails to the shifting political winds and by trying to ingratiate themselves with everybody. This is no setting for medical officers of health, who must fall back, at times, upon the police power to enforce requirements urgently needed for the control of disease, at the risk of offending some local political magnate who has the power to wreck their careers. Here is a very serious weakness in our system, and one which in the past has certainly barred many able men from this field, and admitted only those who were willing to take what most of us would regard as staggering risks with their professional future. The situation is one which can only be remedied by enlightened public opinion, and though the physicians as a body may be of assistance in shaping this opinion, they cannot lead where public opinion is not prepared to follow.

Another profound weakness in our provision for the care and oversight of the public health is our persistent unwillingness to appropriate sums of money sufficient to do the work as it ought to be done. It has been estimated that a reasonably satisfactory staff and organization for the care and oversight of the public health could be provided for about $1.00 per capita of the population. Recent surveys tend to show, that in cities of 100,000, or more, the average appropriation for such purposes varies from sixty-five to eighty cents, whereas in the rural districts the appropriations are in the neighborhood of thirty-five cents.[1] The disinterested observer might readily take the view that such niggardly appropriations were sufficient evidence that, in general terms, the people of this country did not care enough about providing for a satisfactory public health organization to pay for it, and consequently were prepared to get along without it. This conclusion, however, would involve the assumption that any such conscious state of mind exists. It is not the result of intent, but the result of mere carelessness which can probably be remedied only by steady pressure of an educational type. That such pressure has been exercised with considerable benefit, a survey of the progress of the last quarter century will show, and there is no reason for discouragement on the part of those who have spent their lives in moving this problem forward, at what seems to them a snail's pace. They have, I believe, laid the foundation for what may well prove to be considerably more rapid progress in the future. There is evidence, though perhaps observable only by the optimist, that we are approaching the point where we shall be willing to take the care of the public health out of politics, and put it upon a self-respecting basis.

Preventive Medicine for the Individual

It will be possible only to touch upon a few points in this large field, as a method of indicating lines of development which may profitably be considered in sizing up the whole problem.

Child Health Program

Supervision of child health is a field which, until the relatively recent past, has been much neglected in this country. In many European countries provisions have existed for a long time, and such supervision is often better than ours. On the other hand, there is clear evidence that during the last one or two decades public opinion has been considerably stimulated, as shown by the steady growth of the attempts at school health programs. The provision of medical officers employed by local school units to inspect school children has grown relatively rapidly, though it is still far from being complete or satisfactory the country over.

Unfortunately, there have arisen rather serious differences of opinion between the public, as represented by the school authorities, and the medical profession as represented by the local organizations. On many occasions the medical profession has opposed the development of these programs on the ground that such school inspection was likely to be carried over into the field of treatment, thus depriving the private practitioner of his legitimate field. To go into this discussion, and do it any justice, would require more time than can properly be devoted to it. There are of course two sides. The school authorities, representing the public, are likely to see only one phase of the problem. It is quite impossible to draw a sharp line between the children of parents who are amply able to have their children cared for by private practitioners and those who, if simply advised that medical treatment is desirable, will neglect it because they are unable to pay for it. In some instances, at least, this skirmish between the public and the profession has resulted to the disadvantage of the child.

That such programs should be developed by joint conferences between the public, as represented by the school authorities, and the physicians, as represented by their appointed officers, seems perfectly clear. Here, as in a good many other debatable fields in the development of health service, the profession has lacked something, both of leadership, and of open-mindedness, which will prove very essential in the future development of a well-rounded program.

In the development of school health inspection lies the most certain method of developing an enlightened opinion in regard to all forms of immunization against preventable disease. Our school system is, on the whole, so complete that it is possible to ascertain the extent to which such immunization has been carried out, and to provide the proper machinery for the immunization of practically the whole population, limited only by the extent to which the public can be kept advised of the point to which scientific fact has advanced. There is probably no other point in the whole field of preventive medicine at which a concentrated attack, made by people qualified to instruct the public in the certain facts of the prevention of disease, can be made to bring such satisfactory results. The medical profession will be well advised to give more attention to the possibility of education here.

In the same way, through a school health program, the very widespread neglect of dentistry can be attacked. All of the recent studies of the health of school children indicate neglect of dental hygiene and care—this in the face of the fact that the United States is better supplied with well-trained dentists than any country in the world.

Surprisingly enough, however, there are some indications that, unlike the situation in the general practice of medicine, the supply of dentists would be inadequate to carry out a really thorough-going program. If this be true, it will be well to accompany the education of the public in the necessity for dental care with a careful survey of the sources of supply of dental practitioners.

Preventive Medicine for the Adult

One of the important fields of preventive medicine for the adult is that of the further extension of dental prophylaxis and dental care. More and more, as time goes on, the conviction grows that neglected teeth are a not inconsiderable factor in a variety of medical disabilities, and though we have probably led the world in the development of dentistry, we are still considerably short of having convinced the public of its value in the long run. There are still too many people whose whole conception of the province of dentistry is the alleviation of a toothache.

Periodic Health Examinations

I quite recognize that in discussing periodic health examinations one invades a highly controversial field. The evidence of the possible value of such examinations was first put forward, I believe, by the great insurance companies, who came to the opinion, as the result of some check upon the holders of their policies, that periodic examinations were of value, not only to the company, but to the individual. The conception of a regular inventory of the health of an individual is most attractive, and, at least on the face of it, would seem free from serious objection, other than the notorious difficulty of persuading people that it was worth while. The proposition that the individual should periodically be examined by his regular physician, more frequently in the first ten years of life, less frequently during the next twenty or thirty years, and again more frequently as the human machine begins to show evidence of wear and tear, is delightful in its simplicity.

In practice, however, difficulties appear. Any conscientious physician who has undertaken to make a thoroughly complete survey of an individual will recognize at once that the limitations of a single physi cian, even though he have access to the various devices which science has put at his command, are very real. In the first place, he will be faced with some very difficult estimates as to the psychology of his patient, and will have to treat very warily those introspective individuals for whom slight warning tends to look like a death sentence. Again, he will have the gravest difficulties in knowing how far his study should go. Can he be quite sure of his own judgment in regard to the advice which he should give, for instance, in regard to a pair of shopworn tonsils which may or may not be loaded with dynamite? In the presence of a middle-aged patient of either sex with what years ago used to be called "dyspepsia," will he be justified in guessing that the patient has no organic disease concealed beneath his belt, or must he submit the patient to a complete study with barium, fluoroscope, X ray, gall-bladder dye, diluted cream, and all the paraphernalia of a complete gastro-intestinal examination? If he choose the former horn of the dilemma, and the patient proves within a few years to harbor gallstones which some surgeon thinks should be the property of the pathologist, how will he justify his oversight? If, on the other hand, having advised a complete examination and having found nothing, will he have endeared himself to his patient when the bill comes in? Or, suppose the case of a somewhat younger patient who, having perchance treated his body as he would not dare to have treated his dog, is found to have, upon examination of the chest, some "questionable" areas in the lung. Shall he insist upon a thorough X ray study of the chest, and having done so will he, himself, feel confident that he can assure his patient as to the possibility of future developments? Or, take, perhaps, one of the most common stumbling-blocks in the field of diagnosis, a lady of uncertain age apparently addicted to the habit of abdominal pain. His superficial examination shows no evidence of abnormality. How shall he proceed? Will he be justified in relying implicitly upon the findings of such an examination, or must he leave no stone unturned in order that, by the process of elimination, he may assure the lady that the pain is not "of organic origin"—whatever that may mean? In the former case he runs the risk of overlooking some grave lesion which may in fact threaten life. In the latter case he runs the risk of calling her attention so sharply to her internal machinery that, when the smoke clears away, he has left her worse off than when she started.

The situation is a veritable Scylla and Charybdis, and though I am aware that there is much exalted opinion to the effect that the well-trained general practitioner can carry out an examination, as the result of which he can advise his patient, my own experience leaves me in the gravest doubts as to the correctness of this view. It will be possible, of course, to determine by such an examination the presence or absence of obvious abnormality, but most abnormality, in its early stages, is not obvious. The whole theory of the periodic examination is that it shall discover things which are very far from obvious, and certain it is, that if we are to limit its usefulness to the obvious, we shall not include any very early discovery of disease, and shall lose much of its assumed value. Personally, I am unable to convince myself that an examination which is thoroughly satisfactory—and I am not prepared to advise anything else—can be accomplished by any single physician, even though the facilities which are at his command are pretty extensive. Some attempts in this field went far to convince me that, at least, a "team" of some capacity, including specialists in at least four fields besides that of general medical diagnosis, is likely to be required if the job is to be properly done. Furthermore, when the component members of this team have each had their say, it will require a long-headed person to assess the situation and to be quite sure that, when he delivers the opinion of the group, he actually stresses those things which ought to be stressed, and minimizes those things which may be more apparent to the patient and more likely to disturb his sleep than his bodily health. A periodic examination, performed as above suggested, will be a costly business. If we are to insist upon thoroughness, periodic health examinations will not be applicable to a large section of the population. If we do not insist upon it, I feebly suggest that we are quite as likely to do harm as good, and sin, either by commission or omission. In a word, much as I would like to espouse enthusiastically the cause of the periodic health examination as carried out by the careful, conscientious general practitioner, it appears to me so open to possible error as to be of very doubtful utility.

Personnel

THE PRIVATE PRACTITIONER

During the period in which the practice of medicine has changed from a relatively simple to a highly complicated business, other economic changes have been going on, more or less in the opposite direction. Thus, the tendencies in industry have been from complication to simplification, and the era of quantity production ushered in by the World War has taken a strong hold upon our imagination. Perhaps also the War, itself, gave rise to the view that it might be possible to deal with human illness by pretty wholesale methods. Such, of course, was and is inevitably the practice of war, but it is not, and I suspect can never be, the practice of peace. The difference is fundamental. In war the individual hardly exists. In peace, at least in our theory of democracy, the whole basis of our rather loose method of government is based upon the assumption that the largest measure of individual freedom should be given. Though it may well be that we shall come to doubt the extent to which this theory is wholly applicable to the increasingly complicated business of national government, we shall, I think, never arrive at the point where we doubt that the care of illness, as a general proposition, must remain a highly individual matter. This statement is not necessarily out of line with the fact that in the presence of grave epidemic disease the individual, of necessity, must be disregarded, nor is the statement necessarily invalidated by the fact that where, for reasons of economy, large numbers of individuals are brought together under institutional care, some loss of individuality may be inevitable. The fundamental fact remains that, as a general rule, the relation between physician and patient must be a personal one.

Such a relationship was more or less a matter of course at the earlier day when knowledge of disease was rather rudimentary, and almost every practitioner could be regarded as reasonably capable of representing the whole field. That day has gone beyond recall, and as has already been indicated, the mass of detailed knowledge, and the rapidity with which new knowledge becomes available, have required great and permanent subdivision, in the interests of accurate diagnosis—which must ever underlie effective treatment. Though this may seem elementary, and not requiring further elaboration, there remains, not only in the mind of the public, but curiously enough in the minds of many members of the profession, an extraordinary failure to grasp this fact, and we still hear much regarding the importance of returning "the old family doctor" to his original position. As well might one attempt to resurrect the Dodo. The conditions, under which his great place in the community existed, have ceased to exist. It is as futile to attempt to resurrect him as to set back the hands of the clock.

Of course, this does not mean that there is to be an end of what one might characterize as the "generalist" as compared with the "specialist." Such a conclusion would be violently untrue. There is, and, as far as one can foresee, must continue to be a large group, probably constituting a majority of the medical profession, who do not hold themselves out as specialists, who do not pretend to be familiar with the more intricate and more difficult methods of diagnosis or with the application of the newest and, sometimes, most complicated methods of treatment. These "generalists," who perhaps should be called the general practitioners, must have a broad and comprehensive view based upon a fundamental medical training, and enhanced by daily contact with varieties of ailments. On the other hand, unless we are to fail to utilize the broad advances of modern medicine, the general practitioner, emphatically, cannot stand alone. It is at least suggested that the greatest weakness of the present offering of medical service, not only in this country, but elsewhere, is the lack of close, intimate, and, probably, daily contact between the general practitioner and specialists in various fields. Furthermore, not only must this contact with his more specialized brethren be frequent and intimate, but the general practitioner must have at his immediate command all of the more common methods of laboratory diagnosis. These even in his younger days will probably be beyond his individual power to carry out; but if such be not the case at first, as new methods of laboratory tests are developed, he will soon come to have only a bowing acquaintance with their actual performance. If, however, he allows himself to settle into the comfortable, but inefficient, view that a few laboratory tests, such as simple examinations of blood and urine, will enable him to offer a first-class article of service, he will soon find himself attempting to offer to his patients a brand of medicine so outworn and shoddy as not to be worth the price. I suggest, therefore, that an intimate and enlarging contact between the general practitioner, the laboratory, and the specialist is essential to good modern practice of medicine. As time goes on, it is likely to become more rather than less important.

There is a dogma which runs like a master thread through many of the discussions of the general practitioner's place in the scheme of modern medicine. That it has behind it abundant authority is at least suggested by its frequent repetition, and apparently general acceptance. It runs somewhat as follows: "The general practitioner, with only such equipment as he can have in his office, is capable of diagnosing and treating satisfactorily from 80 to 90 per cent of illness." From this dogma I feel required to dissent, since it appears to me to clothe this overworked man with powers quite beyond the capacity of the human mind. One must assume that underlying this dogma there is the understanding that no treatment worthy of the name, or for which remuneration should be asked, can be accomplished without a diagnosis, or at least without every reasonable attempt to come to one. Now, if it is alleged that with his meager equipment and his probable, or inevitable, lack of sufficient time to make searching investigation of many cases, he is to succeed in making a correct diagnosis in 80 per cent, then he is being clothed with an accuracy which is certainly quite beyond his more specialized brethren. That he will of necessity see a large number of cases of trivial illness in which accurate diagnosis is unimportant, because the patient will certainly recover before a diagnosis is made, may readily be admitted. This, however, does not ease the requirement for accuracy. No one can foresee at what moment an apparently trivial ailment may turn out to be the earlier manifestation of some very serious condition. It has been repeatedly stated, without serious dissent, that it is in the earlier stages of serious conditions that accurate diagnosis is most likely to lead to effective treatment. The dogma appears to me to run serious danger of encouraging both physician and public to believe that a rather sketchy examination, without the application of searching tests, will avoid the numerous pitfalls.

Moreover, the estimates suggested above appear to me to overlook very large fields of special knowledge which have already withdrawn some conditions from the field of the general practitioner, are at the present time withdrawing others, and bid fair, as time goes on, to make still further subtractions. Without laying claim to highly special knowledge, it may at least be suggested that there are relatively few diseases of the eye for which the general practitioner can supply the necessary diagnosis and treatment. In the other fields of the special senses—the ear, the nose and throat—modern specialization has carried many of these problems out of the field of the general practitioner and into the purview of the specialist. Again, there are many conditions involving disease of heart or lungs, particularly the earlier manifestations of pulmonary tuberculosis and of heart disease, in which the general practitioner, to say the least, will be put to it to come to an opinion sufficiently accurate to warrant his expecting the patient to follow his advice. The care and feeding of children have altered and advanced pretty rapidly in the last fifteen years. Are those who support the dogma prepared to assert that the average general practitioner is a competent pediatrician? Where shall one draw the line between major and minor surgery. The latter is commonly listed as within the capacity of the general practitioner. In several recently prepared lists of fields, which under the dogma, the general practitioner is expected to cover, I see listed infections and infected wounds, and my mind slips back to the many tragedies of crippled hands as the result of failure to recognize and treat in major and not in minor fashion apparently trivial infections in this region. One is almost tempted to suggest that it were better that the general practitioner delve in the mysteries of abdominal surgery than in the complications of infections of the palmar space. In the one case, perchance, he may lose his patient, but in the other he will be faced by a man whose earning capacity has been cut in two by a crippled right hand.

Turning now to a field with which I have more personal familiarity, I do not hesitate to suggest that there are few if any diseases of the genito-urinary tract, of either sex and at any age, which can today be satisfactorily diagnosed and treated by the general practitioner without constant assistance from the laboratory and the specialist. In a somewhat kindred field, that of so-called—and often miscalled—venereal disease, it would be a bold man who would assert that these conditions can be satisfactorily diagnosed and treated except by those with much more than average knowledge and training. Finally, attention may be called to the large and growing field of disease or dislocation of the nervous system. Here, even the expert travels on treacherous ground. Accurate diagnosis can often be based only upon the most rigid exclusion. The enormous variety of clinical pictures which may be produced by patients waging an unequal combat between a mad world and an unstable nervous system, acquired from antiquity, literally beggars description. The particulars in my bill of complaint could be augmented almost indefinitely. The dogma does not seem to me to rest upon the facts, and I must therefore dissent from it.

The difficulty, as I see it, lies in the fact that, under the present setup, the speed of change has left the general practitioner in an altogether too isolated position. This isolation is not of his making, and has come about partly as a matter of pace, and partly as a matter of economic change. Under our present plan, it is commonly true that only in his earlier years has the general practitioner a sufficient amount of time to study his patients with the thoroughness and resourcefulness which, in those days, he is well equipped to give. As time goes on, he becomes progressively less well equipped and, unfortunately, has less time at his disposal. The well-equipped younger man spends half his time waiting for patients. The less well-equipped older man is driven by sheer necessity to snap diagnosis, hasty treatment, neglect of laboratory studies, with which he may have not even a bowing acquaintance. He is caught in the dilemma that unless he sees and treats a large number of individuals, he may be unable to pay his monthly bills. Such a setup does not encourage searching investigation. It does not encourage the request for assistance and advice from specially qualified colleagues, since both of these cut directly athwart his too precarious income. Every special examination, every consultation, stands at least a chance of diminishing rather than increasing his income, though it would undoubtedly increase and not diminish the value of the service which he offered. This situation appears to me to lie at the root of many of the difficulties of modern practice, and to be the prime factor in the apparently progressive commercialization of modern medical practice. If, instead of perpetuating the dogma that the isolated general practitioner can care for 80 per cent of disease, we would give attention to the possibilities of bringing to his assistance the laboratory and the consultant, without at the same time menacing his livelihood, success would be more likely to attend our efforts. This is, of course, but another way of saying that the day of the isolated individual in the practice of medicine, whether he be generalist or specialist, is approaching its close, if indeed it has not already reached it.

When one attempts to extend the picture and to talk about the importance of reëstablishing the place of the family physician, the matter becomes even more complicated. In the first place, the picture of the family physician, which we most readily call to mind, is based upon the assumption that he will have the care and oversight of a family group over a considerable period of years. This was undoubtedly true fifty years ago, but the development of modern industry, with its tendencies toward concentration and then dispersion, and, probably more important, the extraordinary development of means of transportation, have rendered this conception largely sterile. The family is ceasing, I fear, to be the unit of medical practice, and we must rather turn to the individual to take its place. However, this will not authorize us to disregard the desirability, which is obvious, of a physician's dealing with a family group to as large an extent as possible. I suggest, however, that in the family group the problem is even more beyond his capacity than in the case of the individual.

All of this appears to me to point in one direction: that of relieving the isolation of the general practitioner both as regards the modern laboratory methods of diagnosis and increased contact with consultants and specialists.

THE SPECIALISTS

Having discussed the difficult position of the general practitioner in the present scheme of health service, attention must now be called to the position of the specialist. The extent to which specialization has become an essential part of the modern practice of medicine has already been indicated. Here, the problem is to point out the extent, if any, to which the development of specialization has departed from sound lines, and to indicate methods of better integration. It is frequently said, and with undoubted truth, that the proportion of specialists in the United States is clearly in excess of that to be found in other countries. It is also frequently suggested that this proportion is unnecessarily large—but one proposition does not necessarily follow upon the other. As far as my own experience warrants a conclusion, it appears quite certain that the best development of medical service *in this country* will require a larger proportion of specialists than is at present the case elsewhere. As before suggested, I feel quite confident that the American people are going to expect an amount of special care and special knowledge which is neither expected nor provided elsewhere. This I do not believe to be an extravagance, but rather think it an indication that we can, if we think wisely and clearly, provide ourselves with a better medical service than exists in any other country.

I do not for a moment mean to suggest that at the present time there are not in this country an excessive number of physicians who hold themselves out as having special qualifications. It will be remembered that there is considerable evidence tending to show that something approaching one-half of the physicians in this country have specialized their work to at least some extent. The figure commonly given for Germany and Great Britain more nearly approaches one-third. I am inclined to suggest that the appropriate figure for this country will be below our present one, but above that of any other country.

The problem in regard to specialists appear to me to be a dual one. If I am right in my postulate that we can use to advantage a higher percentage of physicians with special qualifications, it is essential that they should be brought in much more intimate contact with the general practitioner than is possible under our present system. Such an integration is prevented, at the present time, largely by financial obstacles. The specialist can carry on satisfactorily by revolving in a relatively narrow orbit. It is not to his financial advantage to enlarge this orbit, and thereby consume more time in moving about and, in all probability, have to accept lower fees.

Here again we come back to the frequently intruding and troublesome problem of the relation between the fees of the general practitioner and those of the specialist. The prevalent and destructive practices carried on under the general heading of fee-splitting have arisen in this way, and as already indicated, are in fact human, though improper, outcries against an inequitable division. In some income groups the problem must almost certainly be solved by some form of informal grouping of general practitioners and specialists, by which the service of the whole group, as needed, may become available for a single fee, this fee to be apportioned by agreement. This need not involve the formalities of group practice, as ordinarily considered, but a much more informal plan is, I believe, feasible—particularly in the smaller centers of population. Perhaps it can be best achieved through the medium of the hospital, as is now actually being done in various experiments. The greater the extent to which such groups can be kept informal, and more or less constantly changing, the less open they will be to the accidents of personal collisions which are inherent in more rigid grouping. The underlying principle appears to me to be that of the joint fee, entitling the patient to a variety of service without the present difficulty inherent in multiple special fees. The solution of such problems requires ingenuity, good temper, and an abiding determination to resist commercialization. These qualities are essential in the execution of any satisfactory plan for improved health service, and will test the extent to which physicians are able to maintain a professional status and shake off the incubus of commercialization.

The other important requirement in working out the proper proportion and appropriate distribution of specialists is a satisfactory plan for their education. At the present time it is probably true that the majority of those physicians, regarded as specialists both by the profession and by the public, have become specialists without an adequate training, for the very good reason that such adequate training could not be provided. Even at the present time it may fairly be doubted whether the country is fully equipped to provide the essential preliminary training which would generally be accepted by the profession as adequate. Most of our attention in the last twenty years has been centered upon the improvement of undergraduate medical education. Though the education of graduates in special fields has gone steadily forward, it still lacks in concreteness and in organization. That the profession is aware of this need is evidenced by the growing tendency to set up special groups having for their purpose the defining of the qualifications necessary for specialists in the various fields. This process is still far from complete, but is going steadily forward.

However, an essential part of the movement is the increased appreciation by educational institutions of the importance of this development. Undergraduate medical education has come almost wholly under the purview of the Universities. Graduate education at the present time is much less satisfactorily managed. Undoubtedly the great majority of well-trained specialists in this country today have come by their training as the result of prolonged residency in well-equipped hospitals, only a modicum of which are under university control. It is not intended to suggest that it will be wise or possible to concentrate the graduate education in a similar manner to that which has been carried out in the undergraduate field, but it *is* intended to suggest that the groups of specialists in this country who are now engaged in studying and planning for the necessary qualifications, should begin to see to it that all of the hospital establishments capable of offering satisfactory training in the graduate field should be drawn together by common interest and mutual understanding.

The Adequate Supply of Physicians

Even the most cursory study of the number of physicians in this country, as compared with those of any of the other countries, will show that the number is importantly higher in relation to the population. More or less implicit, however, in the frequent statements of the large number is the implication that the number is increasing in relation to the population. This is not true. (See p. 36.) The number is decreasing somewhat, and will apparently continue to decrease, though slowly, until about 1945. There seems therefore to be no need for extraordinary alarm in regard to the fact of numbers. It is important however to make some attempt to estimate whether this number, though clearly in excess of the proportion to be found elsewhere, is in excess of the number which could be used if medical

MEDICAL NEEDS IN THE UNITED STATES 199

service were more widely and equitably distributed. If it should be assumed that we propose to continue the present very uneven and inequitable offering of medical service, then the number is excessive, and we might as well face that fact. If, on the other hand, we are shocked by the very large number of persons in this country, who, at the present time, are perfectly obviously in need of medical service which they do not receive because they cannot afford it, then we need not be too precipitate in attempting to cut down our numbers, and thus insure ourselves against proper care of the sick.

I cannot avoid the conclusion already suggested that we cannot order our house by the medical equipment regarded as suitable for other people. There is much testimony, and I think some evidence, tending to show that we are pretty sensitive in regard to need when the case has been carefully and wisely presented. I am convinced that we are generous, on the whole, and desire a setup under which we can honestly say that adequate care is being supplied, or is within the reach of everyone. That this can be done with the proportion of physicians per capita now actually at work in other countries, I do not believe. Until, therefore, we have squarely faced our facts, have recognized that there is much need for service which is not being supplied, and have satisfied ourselves that this actually can be delivered by a smaller number of physicians than those now in practice in this country, we shall, I think, do well to move slowly in the direction of decreasing the number of doctors.[2] It is desirable that some careful estimate should be made of the optimum number of physicians of both general and special training. This is necessary to any comprehensive plan, and no thoroughgoing social organization can afford to disregard it.

DISTRIBUTION OF PHYSICIANS

Though there is clearly great difference of opinion as to the proper number of physicians necessary for a satisfactory health service, there can be no doubt that, whether or not the present number of physicians is in excess of the requirement, the distribution of physicians is gravely faulty. This has been becoming more evident with the progressive movement of population from rural to urban districts, but it was not until about 1924 that attention was sharply called to this fact. It was widely asserted, at that time, that the number of physicians in the United States was insufficient, and various groups of organized labor went on record as advising a considerable increase in physicians. More careful study of the facts, however, at once revealed that the number of physicians in the country was entirely adequate, and that the difficulty to which attention was being called was not due to a lack of physicians, but to an alteration in their distribution. At about the same time, attention was called to the fact that there was a considerable and increasing number of towns, which in the past had been able to support one or more physicians, which were without a physician. Discussion of this situation has already been undertaken in Chapter III, and therefore will not be repeated here. The causes are almost purely economic, and very definitely related to the problem of competition.

Another very important factor, if one acts upon the assumption that adequate medical service should be available everywhere, is the improbability, or impossibility, that in a sparsely settled area a practitioner—or even two or three practitioners—could offer a grade of medical service which is as good as the public demands, or anywhere near as good as they are entitled to receive. At the moment, however, we are concerned with the indubitable fact of faulty distribution. There is no reason to believe that this distribution will alter for the better, as long as the present pattern of medical service continues. The situation at present is one under which a good grade of medicine, as judged by present standards, cannot be offered because it cannot be paid for. Moreover, no alteration is to be expected as the result of any fiat method. Physicians will go where they can practice medicine at a satisfactory standard, and where they can receive a reasonable compensation. Such a satisfactory standard may be judged to require facilities for proper hospitalization of patients and reasonable access to laboratory facilities and consultants. The method used under the Highlands and Islands Service in Scotland has undoubtedly improved the service by keeping general practitioners in regions where they could not otherwise have earned a living. It is not satisfactory, however, if medical service is to attain the standard above suggested and bring within the reach of the patients the facilities of modern medicine. The Province of Saskatchewan in Canada has been experimenting, of late years, with the employment of municipal doctors under a plan which guarantees the physician a satisfactory income. This is also open to the criticism of lack of sufficiently complete service. To my mind, a more interesting and promising experiment is the plan which has been utilized to a smaller extent by the Ross-Loos Clinic in Los Angeles. This group has as members of its staff a number of physicians living in the surrounding semirural districts. Under this system they have at their disposal the facilities and special service of the clinic. I am told that there are other clinic groups in the country which have been working informally on similar plans, and I am hopeful that further trial will take place.

Nurses

Clearly a well-balanced health service cannot go far without a well-balanced nursing service; the development of medical and nursing service must obviously be more or less parallel. In regard to the number of nurses, the evidence goes to show that the supply is amply sufficient, and probably excessive. But, it is beyond doubt that a very much larger amount of nursing service could be utilized if the machinery were available to pay for it. This is particularly true in the field of public health nursing, where at the present time the number of nurses is considerably below the optimum number, although about equal to the number that can be utilized under available funds. It thus appears that the situation in regard to nursing is similar to, though not identical with, that apparent in regard to physicians, namely, faulty distribution and inadequate finance.

Dentists

Though it is probably true that the available number of dentists in this country is in excess of that available elsewhere, and while it is certainly true that on the average their equipment for practice is excellent, it is by no means clear that the number of dentists is sufficient to make available satisfactory health service in this field if their offerings could be utilized to anything approaching the desirable extent. It is only of recent years that any clear appreciation has developed of the real neglect of dental care and its probable effect upon the general health of the community. Various surveys of the defects of school children, as well as of adults, tend to show that dental defects stand very high in the scale. There is evidence to show that regular and satisfactory care would have avoided many of these defects, and that even now they could be remedied to a considerable extent if dental services were readily available wherever needed. The suggestion is therefore ventured that, in relation to the available supply of physicians and nurses, the supply of dentists is considerably lower, and probably below, the number which could be utilized satisfactorily under the present setup.

Hospitals

In comparison with most other countries the supply of hospitals in the United States is reasonably adequate, but, like the other component parts of health service, they are not satisfactorily distributed. Moreover, there is considerable evidence to show that the supply of hospital beds in some fields is inadequate; in other fields and in some localities it is probably in excess of the requirement. Thus, there is ample evidence that hospitals for the care of mental disease, chronic disease, and tuberculosis are below the requirement of present conditions. These are, in great measure, hospitals financed and supported by the public out of taxation. Their bed occupancy is very high, but the total number of patients cared for is relatively low because of the essential chronicity of the conditions. As contrasted with this, some of the larger centers of population have hospital accommodations in private and charitably supported hospitals quite in excess of the demand, and except in times of unusual financial prosperity, the bed occupancy of these hospitals is usually below the optimum. In times of average, or less than average, prosperity the bed occupancy falls importantly below a satisfactory level, and the support of these hospitals becomes difficult. In contrast with this, there are still in this country areas in which hospital accommodations are lacking, insufficient, or located in inaccessible places. The difficulty in regard to the supply of hospital beds for what may be called "state patients" arises, of course, from a failure to grasp the real extent of the problem and the difficulty in providing the money by taxation. However, where hospital accommodations are excessive, the trouble has arisen out of faulty planning. Hospitals frequently have been built without sufficient previous study of the demand, or, still more frequently, built with a capital outlay quite in excess of the income reasonably to be expected. It is probably true that, in our enthusiasm to encourage the building of hospitals, there has been grave lack of consultation with properly equipped experts, and lack of proper study of the demand. The to-be-expected growth of population will take up the present slack, but it is quite certain that the further construction of hospitals ought to be carried on with much more previous study and foresight. To a large extent, the proper distribution of hospitals, particularly in the less thickly settled areas, will have to come to pass by means of the expenditure of public funds, and provision will have to be made, not only for capital expenditures, but for maintenance.

There is another side of the use and development of hospitals which ought at least to be stated here. It may be judged to be fundamental that the hospital is an essenial adjunct to the practice of modern medicine, not only because it gives opportunity for placing the sicker patients actually in the hospital, but because it puts the essential provisions of laboratory and technical services at the disposal of the physician practicing in the neighborhood. An increased and increasing use of hospitals for this purpose seems in the interests of all concerned. It is possible, of course, to develop laboratory facilities apart from the hospital, and there is a very considerable number of commercial laboratories offering this service. Such service does not seem to me nearly so valuable in the development of future plans for health service as that offered by laboratories incorporated in hospitals. The commercial laboratory is not likely to become the gathering place of physicians; the hospital evidently is serving this purpose more and more. That it is performing this function as much as would be desirable is, I think, doubtful, but there is evidence that to an increasing extent physicians are tending to locate their offices in the neighborhood of, or even actually in, hospitals—a development which seems to me of the greatest promise.

Care of the Indigent

Though it used to be said, and was apparently believed to be true, that the two classes in the community which received the best care were the paupers and the millionaires, I have grave doubts of the truth of this assertion. If it ever was true of the indigent, it has ceased to be so, and is today true, if at all, only in the case of serious illness requiring hospitalization and, possibly, operation. Even this is true only in the relatively larger centers of population. That domiciliary visits and home care of a really satisfactory grade have ever been generally available, I doubt. In the large cities the out-patient departments of the large hospitals, and the independent dispensaries, serve an excellent purpose in this field, and there is ample evidence to show that their facilities are tremendously used. They do not, however, offer a satisfactory coverage of the whole field and except in the larger cities, the offerings are quite sketchy. Probably the basic reason for the incompleteness of the service is that it has never received sufficient financial support. In the case of the service offered by the great charity hospitals and, in like manner, by their out-patient departments, it has been maintained at a high level only by the utilization of physicians whose services, as a rule, are unpaid. If the medical service received by the indigent in these great institutions were to be paid for, whether out of public funds or those contributed by benefactors, the present cost of this service would be enormously increased. Such a plan would, I believe, be beneficial in that it would require the public to face the fact that a proper offering of medical service is not likely to be obtained unless they are prepared to pay for it. In this field there has been a grave failure, on the part of the community at large, to face the facts. It has been content to continue the habits of an earlier day, under which the services of physicians for hospital work could be obtained without payment because it was almost the only method by which a satisfactory clinical training for the practice of medical specialties could be obtained. With the growth and development of medical education on a sound basis, this situation has been entirely altered, and I am firmly of the opinion that in the near future payment for the services of physicians should be placed upon a basis similar to that of other groups of citizens.

The Low Income Groups

It is intended to include in this bracket that very large group of people who are not, in any sense of the word, indigent, but who to some extent are unable—and to another extent, unwilling—to make the necessary expenditures for satisfactory medical care. The group is evidently not one which should be assisted largely from the public purse; yet it is equally certain that under the present setup, the medical service which they get is often inadequate. What is perhaps worse, the occasional very heavy expense falls upon a relatively small number, seriously damages, and occasionally destroys their economic position. The difficulty faced by this very large number of people is not that of a yearly cost distributed over a long period of time, but the unpredictable, and wholly unprepared for, occasional expense. It seems perfectly certain that for this group some method of spreading the cost is essential. Here will be found, of course, a large number of people who are shiftless and improvident, a still larger number of people who live so close to their financial margin of safety, and struggle so hard to maintain a position somewhat beyond their means that they cannot be expected to make provision for illness on the basis of saving, as ordinarily understood.

There is in this group a very large number of people whose knowledge of the strains and stresses brought about by poor health is wholly insufficient. It may be said that for this group education may solve the problem. I doubt it. At all economic levels people save money for, and buy, those things which are made to look attractive and which are "sold" to them. Illness can never be made to look attractive, and I see no effective method by which it can be sold to them in such a manner as to compete with radios and automobiles, to say nothing of what may be classified as "paint, paper, and whitewash."

It appears inescapable that the problem of these people must be dealt with by some form of group payment. It seems further probable that these payments should not be planned so as to cover the whole cost, but so as to break the back of the tremendous loads with which they are brought to their knees under the present system.

That entirely voluntary provision will work for this group is against general experience, since it will inevitably fail where it is most necessary—in the case of the careless, shiftless, and incompetent. The proposition appears to me to be clear that failure on the part of this group to make some reasonable provision must not be allowed to be visited upon their dependants. The further discussion of this problem will be postponed to a later chapter.

The Medium Income Group

The extreme difficulties of the large section of the population which should be included in the group previously discussed, do not of course bear with the same severity upon the people with better incomes. On the other hand, these people, commonly referred to as people of moderate means, very frequently find themselves in grave financial embarrassment on account of unexpected and severe illness. They are also the group who at the present time guard themselves by use of the insurance principle against many of the other accidents incident to the precarious business of living. These are the people who carry life insurance, who insure against accident and fire, and often insure their automobiles. At the present time they very rarely insure their health, for the very good and sufficient reason that no satisfactory method of doing so has as yet been instituted. For them I do not despair of the employment of the principle of voluntary group prepayment plans. It is quite evident from the experience in Great Britain that to a large and increasing extent they will insure themselves in such a way as to provide hospital accommodations. It seems to me at least probable that for this group the principle of voluntary insurance can be made useful, if proper plans are made for its offering.

XIII

SOME SUGGESTED METHODS OF IMPROVEMENT

The amount and breadth of the discussion of the problem of adjusting medical service to the needs of the population has resulted in the accumulation of a mass of testimony which, though very enlightening, is of necessity confusing. The work of the Committee on the Costs of Medical Care resulted in the production of a large amount of factual evidence of first-class importance. Too frequently, in discussions previous to this report—and even since that time—opinions have been expressed based upon insufficient information, though the evidence was available. On the other hand, many of the questions involved are, and must remain, matters of opinion. But it is of real importance to utilize the very large amount of available evidence which bears directly or indirectly upon these problems. A volume could be devoted to a careful examination of the multitude of suggested methods of approach; to do so might well be a waste of time, and certainly is beyond the scope of this volume. An attempt will be made here to examine some of the possible methods of approach, and weigh their availability.

Insurance

Insurance is a method by which, in many other fields, it has been possible to spread the cost of unusual and unexpected expenditures over a term of years, in such a way that the burden is moderate and bearable. The problem of spreading the cost of medical care—and at the same time providing sufficient income to carry on medical service of high grade—is in some respects similar to that in fields where insurance methods have proved satisfactory. It is therefore obvious that a careful examination must be made of various applied and suggested methods of using this principle. Moreover, there is now available a large amount of experience which is valuable in evaluating the possibilities and difficulties. It is arguable that most of the difficulties and objections have already been developed and that

208 SUGGESTED METHODS OF IMPROVEMENT

a careful study of the field will warrant something approaching definite conclusions as to the possibilities of applying the method. In many of the discussions which have taken place in recent years, the effect of the opinions expressed has been weakened by evidence of lack of knowledge of available information. Very sweeping statements have been made upon both sides which do not appear to me to be warranted by the evidence. On the one side may be placed the quite positive statements of various experts in the economic field to the effect that some form of compulsory insurance will obviously be required,[1] while on the other side has been the frequent assertion—generally from physicians—that compulsory health insurance leads straight to socialism, pauperization, and ruin of the medical profession.[2] I am frank in admitting that it does not seem to me clear that either of these positions is sound, and I feel required, therefore, to review briefly some of the evidence.

VOLUNTARY INSURANCE AGAINST SICKNESS

NATIONAL

Perhaps the outstanding example of voluntary health insurance may be found in Denmark.* The evidence seems sufficient to warrant the conclusion that the workings of this system in Denmark have been advantageous to all concerned. A large percentage of the whole population is embraced in the plan. The quality of medical service appears to be good, and the physicians, a very large proportion of whom are working under the plan, at least to some extent, seem to be satisfied. There is no evidence that the plan has in any way hampered the development of medical science and the contributions of the Danes to medical progress have been noteworthy. It should be noted, however, that the system is not quite voluntary and that there is a left-handed threat involved, in the loss of certain political and social rights of the improvident who may have failed to insure themselves under the system. To this extent, therefore, the system is not strictly voluntary. Some doubt may arise as to whether, without this measure of compulsion, it could have been made as complete as it is at present. Any attempt to draw

* Since this was written, the system in Denmark has been made compulsory, but the value of the example remains.

SUGGESTED METHODS OF IMPROVEMENT

conclusions as to the availability of the method for application in this country must also take account of the very fundamental differences of the problem. Denmark is a small country with a relatively homogeneous population of 3,500,000. The spread between the richest and the poorest is considerably less than that to which we are accustomed here, and the proportion of those properly called indigent is small. Furthermore, politically speaking, Denmark has gone slowly and steadily forward in the direction of socialization to an extent far beyond what is even contemplated here. Finally, there appears to be little of that very unruly element in the population which makes any social experiment for us difficult. We are bound, therefore, to conclude that while voluntary or quasi-voluntary health insurance has been carefully and skillfully established in Denmark, and is furnishing a pretty satisfactory solution to their problems, it is difficult to see how their experience can be of important assistance to us. In other countries where there exist varying degrees of voluntary insurance supervised by the government, there has been, as a rule, a considerable background of medical care on a contract basis by various forms of friendly and coöperative societies. Where such a situation exists, it is relatively simple for the government to take a hand in the supervision of the affairs of the societies, regulate to some extent their charges, and make the necessary contributions from taxation which lead to success. No such situation exists in this country. The development of the Friendly Society, and its prototype in various countries, has made but little progress here. Therefore it may fairly be doubted whether voluntary insurance, supervised and assisted by the government, will be a valuable method of approach here, at least for a long time to come.

VOLUNTARY INSURANCE NOT PARTICIPATED IN BY THE GOVERNMENT

Health insurance by regular life and accident companies.—Interestingly enough, though it might appear that health insurance was an excellent field for the solid, conservative, well-managed insurance companies, they have not played a large part in the solution of the problems which are being considered here. After all, we are concerned chiefly with the delivery of, and payment for, satisfactory medical service to people in the lower income-brackets. This at once limits the field of the insurance company. The risk in general health insurance has been, on the whole, rather unpredictable. The rates at which the companies could afford to offer this insurance, on a basis profitable to themselves, have been relatively high—thus putting it generally beyond the reach of the group with which we are here most concerned. Moreover, such insurance is most likely to be used by the careful, conservative, provident individuals, who constitute an unfortunately small proportion of the population, and are least likely to find themselves in difficulty. At least up to the present time, health insurance of this kind, though in the total a large number of persons have been insured, has not appeared to be a probable solution of the problem.

Various private voluntary plans for partial insurance.—One of the most interesting experiments in this field has been the British Hospital Savings Association. This has developed in Great Britain largely because of the incomplete character of compulsory health insurance under which no provision is made for hospitalization. That hospital costs are an important item will be obvious. Under this plan, persons with incomes below a certain level may obtain at a reasonable rate, from groups of British hospitals, certainty that hospital care will be available in case of serious illness. The rapidity and extent to which this form of insurance has grown in England suggests that it may be a very valuable adjunct to their existing arrangements for partial medical care. Thus, as a supplement to some existing plan, and quite certainly under the conditions in Great Britain, this plan seems assured of an important measure of success. There appear to be no grave objections other than the difficulties which are certain to arise in regularly providing hospital accommodations at the exact moment that they are desired by the insured.

The American hospital insurance plans.—Perhaps stimulated by the discussion which resulted from the publication of the report of the Committee on the Costs of Medical Care, there are developing, at the present time in many parts of this country, plans under which groups of local hospitals undertake to provide hospital care on the basis of a fixed yearly payment. These plans are mentioned here simply to point out that they are important evidence that hospital groups are aware of the importance of the problem and are moving to play their part. Few, if any of them, are in operation, or, if in operation, have not been going long enough to warrant any conclusions as to the soundness of the experiment. They are attempting to offer insurance against an important item in medical costs. They will encounter, of course, the difficulties and complications incident to obtaining the coöperation of large groups. Also, in some parts of the country they have already encountered difficulties flowing from existing statute law providing for oversight of all forms of insurance by the state. There are already some rulings to the effect that these plans do, in fact, constitute insurance, and must come under the supervision of the state insurance authorities. This may or may not prove to be an important obstacle, but serves to illustrate the difficulty encountered by private organizations in an attempt to set up broad plans.

Medical insurance by private groups of physicians.[3]—For a number of years, experiments in offering medical service to lay groups on an insurance basis have been tried by organized groups of physicians in various parts of the country. This is, in some ways, a logical extension of the development of group practice, since a private group, having been developed, is in a position to offer partial or complete medical service without serious disarrangement of its already existing organization. In some instances the groups have been developed largely for the purpose of offering such insurance. One of the outstanding cases of this type is that of the Ross-Loos Clinic in Los Angeles. As has already been pointed out, since 1929 this group has been engaged in a definite form of voluntary health insurance. The evidence seems satisfactorily to show that the service offered has been of good grade. Various adjustments of the fee charged have been necessary, and it is by no means clear that a final figure has been reached. This, however, is a relatively unimportant detail, and the work done by this group appears to warrant the opinion that, at least in large centers of population, organizations of this kind can be conducted successfully, at a cost to the patient which will bring it within the reach of many persons of the lower income-brackets. It appears to me to be a very valuable demonstration, and one which it is in the public interest to continue, and should have the support of the medical profession.

Organizations centering around the county medical societies.— Of late years, a variety of interesting and important experiments have been tried, centering around the organization of the county medical societies. These experiments are certainly important as evidence of attempts at coöperative medical action. They have almost always been set up to cover persons in the low income-brackets— often chiefly, or entirely, those properly regarded as indigent. Probably none of them have been in operation long enough to warrant conclusions in regard to the various types of organization, but they undoubtedly are giving valuable evidence as to this very important method of attack upon the problem. The county medical society has not been, as a rule, a very homogeneous group. As is rather characteristic of all organizations of physicians, it has had difficulty in handling its own members. Physicians are notoriously individualistic; their whole background and training makes them prefer to act as individuals rather than in groups. In many ways such a tendency is probably inherent in their work, since the problems with which they deal—those of illness—must be handled individually in order to be solved successfully. This will increase the difficulty of concerted, carefully planned, and accurately executed action by such groups. Moreover, the membership of a county society has always been a changing one; it is to be hoped that this shifting tendency will not too much disappear. If the medical profession can succeed in delivering a satisfactory article of medical service through the united efforts of organizations such as the county medical societies, it will have gone far to justify its claim of being capable to handle such problems on its own initiative. The whole question is at present in too early a stage of development to warrant conclusions.

ESTIMATE OF THE PROBABLE VALUE OF VOLUNTARY INSURANCE

From these examples of present experiments in voluntary insurance, it is perhaps possible to draw some tentative conclusions. On a national scale, voluntary insurance is at its best in countries of small and homogeneous population. Furthermore, it is best suited to people having stable governments and a relatively advanced

SUGGESTED METHODS OF IMPROVEMENT

position in social progress. It does not appear to offer important assistance in our problems. Voluntary insurance on a private basis, on the face of it, should be a useful method in this country. We are, or at least have been, a nation of individualists, who preferred to do things in our own way, and only as a last resort call upon the government. It further appears to me to be true that a handsome number, and perhaps a handsome proportion, of the people who are menaced by the accident of illness are careful, reasonable, and provident. This would then appear to be an excellent field for the development of various types of voluntary insurance. On the other hand, though the problem has faced us for many years, there is no clear evidence that voluntary insurance has been making great progress. Of late years, and under the scourge of hard times, a great deal more activity has appeared. It frequently has been noted that voluntary insurance plans, set up under government auspices, have very generally led to compulsion. This is of course to be expected, since the government, once having entered into the operation, is under pressure to make it succeed, or to forfeit its mandate. This criticism does not apply to any form of voluntary insurance, not under government auspices. Therefore, it seems perfectly safe to encourage voluntary associations, particularly voluntary associations of physicians, in developing this method to the end that its real limitations may become clear.

Compulsory Health Insurance

The previous discussion of some of the forms of compulsory health insurance will have indicated that, for our purposes, the forms developed in Germany and in Great Britain will be the most interesting examples. In Germany, the service under the government is quite complete, providing not only general medical care, but also laboratory, consultant, and hospital care. On the other hand, the British plan is quite incomplete, since it only provides such care by the general practitioner as he can carry out by office and home visits. In considering the value of these examples, it is important to remember that in both instances they were set up primarily as an attack on the problem of poverty, and not primarily as a method of providing medical service. From this developed a double-headed approach: (1) the attempt to give compensation for time lost through illness and thus relieve poverty, and (2) the attempt to provide medical care to the end that illness be cared for as promptly as possible. No one will deny that both of these objectives are desirable, and perhaps necessary, but they make poor bedfellows. There is no necessary similarity in the measures properly to be taken to compensate people for time lost through illness, and those necessary to care for the health of persons in the same group. Many of the difficulties which have arisen have come from this dual method of attack.

In estimating the effect of compulsory health insurance, two aspects of the question must be remembered. Obviously, the prime purpose is to care for health, but as an important adjunct to this care must be the satisfactory maintenance and development of the body of physicians involved. Compulsory insurance in Germany, on the basis of available evidence, undoubtedly has improved the medical care offered to people in the low income-brackets. It has been periodically broadened to include more and more people, and, particularly of late years—when incomes have fallen seriously—has come to include a large portion of the population. It thus follows that its perpetuation has become an important article of political faith, and attempts to modify or to reorganize it are bound to face serious political objection. Though the question is involved in a mass of contradictory, and probably prejudiced, evidence, it appears to be true that the effect of the plan upon the body of medical practitioners has been unfavorable. Private, competitive medical practice has been very much diminished, and is now the chief source of income for only a modest proportion of the physicians. It is probably conservative to say that this experiment has been pushed to a reasonably logical conclusion, and has resulted in improved medical care, but with objectionable effects upon the body of physicians upon which it depends for its success. To an outside observer it would appear essential that radical reorganization must be undertaken. What form this will take under the present dictatorship cannot be predicted.

As compared with the system of compulsory health insurance in Germany, that in Great Britain has very important differences. The

SUGGESTED METHODS OF IMPROVEMENT

most important perhaps is that the service is only partial. The second is that there has been maintained freedom of choice of physicians and direct negotiation between the representatives of the medical profession and the government. There can be no doubt, I think, that the system has importantly improved the care which the wage-earning class receives to the extent that it is covered by the Insurance Act. Upon this point there appears to be very wide agreement among competent observers. It further appears to be true that the Insurance Act has somewhat increased, and importantly stabilized, the income of the general practitioner in Great Britain. The unsatisfactory workings of contract practice, particularly in the large centers of population, have disappeared. There has been an end of undesirable competition between physicians for these contracts. To this extent, and it is an important one, the Act has served an excellent purpose. Perhaps the most important weakness of the Act is its incompleteness, lacking as it does laboratory, consultant, and hospital factors. These difficulties have been clearly recognized, both by the government and by the medical profession. A most illuminating report from the British Medical Association, in 1930, shows clearly that they recognized the desirability for further extension of the Act in the above-mentioned fields. It also demonstrated very clearly the extent to which the profession, as represented by the British Medical Association, was able to grasp the extremely complicated questions involved, and deal with them in a thoroughly statesmanlike manner. On the whole, the relation between the British Medical Association and the Ministry of Health has been one of the most encouraging developments in a field where quarrel and disagreement have been so common. Where the government and the experts involved can keep their discussions on such a high plane, there appears to me to be every reason to expect a satisfactory solution. The profession in this country has, I think, something to learn from a careful reading of the discussions between these two parties.

Other difficulties which have developed under the Act center around two provisions—one is the combination of the monetary benefit and medical benefit, the other is the relation to the Act of the Approved Societies. The attempt in the Act to combine monetary compensation and medical benefit has had the undesirable effect of placing the physician working under the Act in a difficult, at times impossible, position. Obviously the prime duty of the physician is to care for his patient with a view to restoring him to full working capacity. If an attempt is made to combine with this the function of a referee upon whom devolves the responsibility for deciding how long monetary benefit shall be paid, the physician is at once awkwardly placed. The other difficulty arises in the extent to which the Approved Societies are interposed, or interpose themselves, between the physician and the patient. This difficulty of course has been much more serious in Germany where the power of the *Krankenkassen* has been much greater. In Great Britain it has been less serious, but continually crops up where the funds of the societies are such that they can afford to contribute benefits not provided under the Act. Here the layman who holds the purse strings is called upon to give an opinion upon a purely medical question and there is certain to arise not only irritation, but inefficiency. These difficulties are avoidable. Certainly, they could be avoided where any fresh attempt was made to set up compulsory insurance. That they should be avoided in any original setup must be evident, since their removal later is fraught with the possibility of political conflict, and the relative improbability that the questions at issue will receive wholly dispassionate consideration.

We must now attempt some estimate of the possible applicability of any plan of compulsory health insurance in this country. This is necessary because, as above suggested, there are considerable groups of wise and important people who believe that such an experiment should be made, and at once. Interestingly enough, the movement for legislative enactment of compulsory health insurance was most active from 1914-1920. The movement apparently then died down. At that time it certainly did not have the support, and in fact did have the opposition, of organized labor. There is evidence that further proposals along this line will be made during the next few years, and it is of the first importance that they should be discussed fully, temperately, and with a reasonable appreciation of the conditions under which such experiments have been made in other countries, as well as the conditions which such legislation will have

SUGGESTED METHODS OF IMPROVEMENT

to face here. It should at once be apparent that the political, as well as the social conditions in this country, are quite dissimilar to those which exist in countries where such experiments have had long and somewhat satisfactory trials. In the first place, it is inherent in our problem that there are forty-eight different states, and unless it is proposed to set up an organization for compulsory health insurance on a national basis, we must face the fact of the great differences in population, income, and social problems in the different states. From this it follows that the possibility of success will vary greatly, even though it be concluded that there are some states in which such an experiment could wisely be tried. However, a trial by some favorably situated states would be an interesting experiment.

It is next important to consider the necessary size of the unit of population as a satisfactory basis for such an experiment. Obviously, as I think, there are states in the union in which the population is too small and the resources inadequate to give such an experiment even a chance of success. I do not know of any controlling opinion as to the number of people necessary for a successful, or possibly successful, attempt. On the other hand, it must be clear that if the law is to be drawn on the basis of the employed population—that is to say the industrial population—there must be a sufficient number of large and stable industries employing a large and relatively stable group of employees. Experiments in other countries appear to me to show clearly that one of the rocks upon which such experiments are most likely to splinter is failure to accumulate sufficient reserves in reasonably good times. A plan which may work successfully in average times will break down disastrously when business diminishes, wages fall, and unemployment increases. But, that is precisely the time at which large contributions must be readily available. It is precisely the time at which labor and industry are least able to make their contributions, and when the contribution of the state must be greatly increased. Obviously, the contribution of the state can hardly be expected to come from current taxes, but must inevitably come from reserves set aside during favorable periods. If the population which it is proposed to insure is not sufficient to make a considerable contribution to such reserves, and if the population of the state cannot readily contribute, in the form of taxes, amounts which will enable large reserves to be accumulated, then the whole thing will fall to the ground.

If such an act proposes to insure people not engaged in industry, the contribution by the state must be proportionately increased, since the amount ordinarily contributed by industry will be lacking. Thus, in states having a large agricultural and a small industrial population, such a plan, of necessity, will involve a considerably larger contribution from the taxpayer. For this reason, states with a sparse population and—as is likely also to be the case—a small income, cannot undertake such insurance, as, quite obviously, they will be unable to operate it.

States with a large industrial population and a smaller agricultural group will be more likely to be able to handle the thing, provided what may be called the "pot" is large enough. Quite certainly, under such an act, the per capita contribution of the employee and the per capita contribution of the business for the employee must be relatively small. Now, unless the total number to be covered by such insurance is large, the accumulation of a satisfactory reserve will become difficult or impossible. I should doubt whether such an experiment could be set up, with any probability of success, in a unit where there were less than one and a half million people covered by the act.

The next difficulty which is likely to intrude itself is that of mobility of population and mobility of business. Where the act includes the whole country, if public opinion backs it, the people concerned must of necessity acquiesce. Such a situation, however, does not occur if insurance is set up with the state as the unit. If, for example, the contribution asked from the employee should seem to him burdensome, there is nothing to prevent him from leaving the state. Though business is perhaps less movable than labor, the same situation could readily occur and should the charges against industry appear oppressive, business would undoubtedly move out. These contingencies are beyond the control of a single state, and therefore to a considerable extent handicap any such experiment at the outset.

Finally, we must face the necessary and probable consequences of our form of government and our types of political organization. It appears to me clear that the world's experience has shown that success in such ventures can only be achieved where the operation of the act is in the hands of people with experience and permanency of tenure. As far as I am aware, all of the successful experiments in Europe have been achieved by personnel with relative security. For our purposes, I think the best evidence is the success of compulsory insurance in Great Britain. Even the most cursory examination of their organization will show that it depends profoundly upon great security of tenure for those people who administer it. Even in Great Britain, many difficulties and disagreements have arisen between the Ministry of Health, the Approved Societies, and the Medical Profession. That they have not proved disastrous is clearly due to the experience gained by those in charge of these operations. To be quite specific, the fact that Sir George Newman, a physician experienced in medical education and public health, has been for many years in charge of this operation for the government appears to me to be one of the most important factors in its success. It seems to me quite inconceivable that anything short of great permanency of tenure can promise any result approaching success. Now, permanency of tenure has been notoriously lacking in our political setup. One of the gravest difficulties with our public health administration, in the states, has been that it has not proved attractive to men of first-class ability, since their whole career depended upon their ability to satisfy their immediate political superiors, who were themselves dependent for their positions upon a changing, ill-informed, and unpredictable public opinion. If our public health service has been unable to attract regularly men of training and ability, it seems unlikely that we shall be able to attract, to a much more complicated and difficult field, men of the calibre essential to success. Let us make no mistake about it. Any form of compulsory health insurance requires for its administration knowledge, wisdom, and patience. These attributes are required on the part of all the parties concerned. The requisite knowledge and experience can be obtained, at least in this country, only by long tenure of office. At the present time, we have no people equipped by actual experience to carry on the work. They must be trained, and they cannot be trained in the shifting sands of state and party politics. At best, these experiments must be based upon accumulating knowledge.

The conditions with which they must deal are less fixed in this country, and therefore less predictable than abroad. For us, the experiment would be more of an experiment. We have here no important background of the Friendly Society type; the employee group has little experience in dealing with medical care provided under such auspices. The above considerations appear to me to show the very grave difficulties which must be faced by compulsory health insurance in this country, particularly if set up by separate states. Our background has prepared us less than has been the case elsewhere. Our political organization is less well suited to the conduct of social and economic experiments. Finally, our units of population are very varied and relatively unstable. One has but to recall the fate of various insurance projects—such as the insurance of deposits in banks—undertaken by various states, to entertain an abiding skepticism as to the probability of success for compulsory health insurance on a state basis. If, and when, it is proposed to set up such an organization on a federal basis, we shall have something else to think about.

Guild Medicine

It might appear unnecessary to discuss the possibility of the development of guild medicine were it not for the fact that such a proposal has been put forward by a distinguished medical educator,[4] and the phrase "guild medicine" has begun to have some standing in communications both from the laity[5] and from the medical profession. At the outset it appears to me to be important to understand what the word "guild" properly means, and to examine to what extent it would be desirable to organize the medical profession in such a way as to resemble anything properly called a guild. This will require some statement of the nature and origin of the guilds.

In their inception, guilds were merely voluntary trade associations. Beginning with the twelfth century they began to develop into monopolies which controlled the trade of a city—or some branch of trade. They were soon acknowledged by the feudal lords and by the governing bodies of the cities, and came to occupy an official position. At this stage they were probably merely an acknowledgement of an existing fact. As time went on, they began to exert considerable influence on municipal government. Somewhat later there developed the craft guilds. As early as 1100, there were a number of them in France, and by the thirteenth century they were common organizations in most cities of northern Europe and of England. These craft guilds constituted essentially privileged bodies. They were based on protectionism and exclusiveness, and represented a system wholly remote from anything which could be called industrial liberty. Their principal aim was to protect their members against competition, not only from other cities, but from their fellow-workers. It thus developed that they secured the independence of their individual members by a very strict subordination of the members to the rules of the guild. No member was allowed to injure another by improving methods of production, and technical progress was regarded as disloyalty. Each guild had power to restrict its membership, and they became monopolies with an increasingly limited membership. By the fourteenth century this tendency to monopoly and privilege had begun to interfere with the public welfare. By the eighteenth century, in England, the guilds lost most of their former prerogatives. Those remaining were definitely abolished by laws of 1818 and 1835. To sum up, therefore, the guild is a self-constituted body which then becomes regularly authorized to carry on a trade or craft as a monopoly, to fix prices, to restrict its membership, and to exercise complete disciplinary control over the group.

I am interested to note that Professor Scammon takes the view that medicine has been—and it appears that he believes it still is—in broad terms, a guild, and that it has had more or less continuous existence for more than five hundred years. I cannot find the evidence that the medical profession, as it has existed during the last century or two, was ever in fact a guild organization. That there was an Apothecaries' Guild and a Barbers' Guild is true, but with the development, during the last hundred years, of what we think of as the physician, in any proper sense of the word, no such organization has existed. In England at the present time, where perhaps such an organization would be most likely to persist, there is nothing approaching a monopoly in the sense in which the word might be used in this country to cover physicians practicing medicine under license from the state. It will be remembered that England has no system of licensure—only one of registration—and that there is no legal restriction of the practice of medicine.

However, these are largely theoretical considerations; the point which I wish to raise is whether or not any form of organization, properly called a guild, would be a sound one for the practice of medicine, and one to be regarded as in the public interest. Guild medicine, properly so-called, would require the establishment of a monopoly. It would further require that this group should have full power to restrict its membership, to fix fees, and to determine the extent to which new discoveries might be utilized in the practice of medicine. The development of the laws regulating medicine in this country, and the general attitude of the public toward the medical profession, does not seem to me to authorize the view that the people would be at all likely to assent to any such organization. Moreover, it does not appear to me that such an organization would be in the public interest, since it would inevitably tend to restrict the number of practitioners, quite irrespective of the rights of the public. It might at any time operate to delay progress; that was, on the whole, one of the most striking attributes of the guild in its palmy days. Finally, it would operate to control prices, and in this way would certainly come into collision with public interest.

That the organization of the medical profession at the present time in no way resembles a guild seems to me perfectly clear. The profession, as such, has no control over the admission of persons to the right to practice medicine, nor over their dismissal in case of breach of the laws regulating medical practice. In fact, we might easily come to the opinion that it would be desirable for the organized medical profession to have more power over its membership. At the present time, medical organizations have the undoubted right to expel physicians from medical societies, but such expulsion in no way operates to curtail the right of such a person to practice medicine, and there are many instances in which physicians, expelled from medical societies for infraction of the rules, have brought suit in the civil courts, alleging damage to their business, and have been upheld.

It is not pertinent, however, to inquire whether it might be desirable to endow the organized and licensed practitioners of medicine with the monopolistic rights and privileges of the guild. Such a situation does not now exist, and there does not appear to me to be any evidence that the temper of public opinion favors any such development. In fact the suggestion that medicine is, or ought to be, a monopoly managed and controlled in the interests of its membership appears wholly at odds with the basic doctrine that the practitioner of medicine in the modern state is a servant of the people and not its master. The whole theory upon which medicine has developed, at least during the last century, follows this doctrine, and to advocate or suggest a doctrine wholly opposed to this relationship would appear to me to be distinctly a backward step. I feel, therefore, that the use of the word "guild" in connection with planning for improvement of the offerings of health service is not only confusing, but may tend to prejudice, to some extent, the case for developments along sound and coöperative lines.

XIV
LAISSEZ FAIRE OR COMPULSION

In attempting to form any opinion as to what changes and adjustments, if any, should be made in the present plans for the offering of medical service, we may follow one of at least three lines:

1. We may do nothing, except to try to make medical service as good from the point of view of education and ethical standards as may be, and then allow nature, so to speak, to take its course.

2. We may experiment with the adoption, with or without alterations, of some plan which has been extensively tried in some other country, and which appears to have worked fairly well there.

3. We may proceed upon the assumption that the situation is sufficiently serious to require action, but that the evidence does not warrant an attempt to transplant, to this country, even the principles of the practices obtaining elsewhere.

The Doctrine of Laissez Faire

Throughout much of the discussion which has gone on during the last five or six years, there has run an undercurrent of the suggestion that change in any important way was undesirable, that the offerings of health service in this country were on the whole good, though by no means perfect, and that any attempt seriously to alter the even tenor of our ways would probably get us into more serious difficulties. In my travels about the country, I have found that this point of view is very commonly held by members of the profession past middle life. I do not find it so commonly held by physicians under forty-five. The attitude of many of the older physicians is fairly accurately portrayed in an article in the *Atlantic Monthly* in 1931. This article was written by a physician of large experience in general practice, and is entitled to serious consideration because of its source. Undoubtedly, it fairly represents the opinions of a large number. One or two quotations may serve to show the general line of thought.

After long and careful pondering of the question, I am convinced that the people of the middle class have themselves to blame for the "unconscionably high" cost of their medical care. By accepting as axiomatic that the value of medical service is in direct proportion to its cost, they have certainly not discouraged medical men from charging all the traffic will bear. The multitude of people newly enriched by the prosperity following the war helped to strengthen this idea. By failing to discriminate between luxury and comfort, the cost of hospitalization is needlessly increased. By accepting without question the creed of the specialist, that the field of medicine is so vast that no one mind can hope to keep up with its progress, they have encouraged specialism and its off-spring, group practice. . . .

The main reason, however, for the plight of the middle class is their unthinking acceptance of that shibboleth of the specialist, "The practice of medicine has become so complex that no one mind can attempt to keep up with its progress." At first thought this sounds plausible, and it has certainly had its effect upon the attitude of the public toward its medical advisers. More than anything else, the universal appeal of this idea has encouraged the overgrowth of specialism. In turn, the cost of medical care to the middle class has advanced in almost direct proportion to the increase of specialists. . . .

"Keeping abreast of medical progress" is not so difficult as the specialist would have us believe. As Doctor Crookshank said in a recent *Forum*, "A vast deal of rubbish has been written about the impossibility of any one man's grasping all the recent advances in medical science. I say 'rubbish,' because real science simplifies and does not confuse; it synthesizes and leads back to first principles, so that men of intelligence and judgment can with ease keep themselves abreast of the best opinion." . . .

The solution of the medical problem of the middle class is, after all, simple. It is for every family to select one physician for its medical adviser. This man should be selected with great care, then trusted as long as he is found worthy of confidence. If the right sort of man is chosen, and knows that he is the absolute guardian of the family health and that he is expected to call in the help of a specialist or a group of specialists when he deems it necessary, he will put forth his best efforts to merit this confidence. His professional pride, combined with a personal interest in his patient, will make him more anxious to get results than any specialist would be.[1]

It will not be necessary to repeat here what has previously been said to the effect that this doctrine does not seem to me to make sense. It is all very well to advise the selection of a family physician, but since the selection must be made without even the vaguest knowledge of the article sought, success does not seem to me likely. Moreover, the statements to the effect that one man can readily keep pace with the progress seem to me sheer nonsense. In practice, I do not see that it works. The general practitioners obviously do not keep really up-to-date. Moreover, at least in many parts of the country, the selection of the specialist by the general practitioner has become a pretty commercial business.

A somewhat similar point of view is voiced by Doctor Moser. Among other things, he says:

> One of the most challenging realizations to the general practitioner is the fact that he must attempt to know something of every disease which afflicts the human body and that consequently he can scarcely excel in any one thing. He must therefore look around and recognize those of his colleagues in every branch of medicine who know more in their particular practice than he. (Excepting always the soul to soul relationship of a family physician and his patient.) It is the duty and the privilege of the general practitioner to seek the advice and help of the specialist in every doubtful case possible. I consider it almost criminal for a physician to continue treating a serious illness alone if he knows another who could possibly aid him if called into consultation. In addition to the direct benefit to the particular patient every such consultation can be a source of knowledge to the physician calling on a specialist for help.
>
> However, the consultant is often at a disadvantage. He may have never seen the patient before, while the family doctor may have studied his patient over a long period of time. The family physician needs sufficient courage to stand up for his convictions until proved wrong.
>
> On the other hand, the family physician should not ask those financially unable to pay for a consultation with an expensive specialist, to undertake such obligations if he believes himself capable of treating the patient, even if such treatment should come under the heading of a specialty.[2]

Doctor Moser appears to recognize, somewhat more clearly than does Doctor Johnson, the real difficulties of grasping the whole field of medicine, in its present development. He leaves himself, as I think, in a rather serious dilemma when he admits that it is "almost criminal for a physician to continue treating a serious illness alone," yet takes the view that financial considerations may make the calling of a consultant impossible. I have already called attention to this dilemma. It seems to me a very real one, partly because I profoundly doubt the dogma in regard to the qualifications of the average general practitioner, partly because I cannot conceive how the public is to identify the general practitioner who has really been able to keep himself abreast of progress. Finally, I am appalled at the proposition that the diagnosis in difficult cases should be allowed to rest upon the accidental finances of the patient.

If this is the best that the older generation of physicians has to offer us, then I believe they have failed to grasp the situation as it appears to the public.

The doctrine of laissez faire has on the whole been supported by the American Medical Association. The Association, through its Editor and Secretary, was rather severe in its criticisms of the *Majority Report* of the Committee on the Costs of Medical Care. They spoke rather unkindly of the men who conducted the investigations, and of the foundations and individuals who financed it. Their general line of reasoning is quite similar to that quoted from Doctor Johnson.

In an editorial appearing in the *Journal of the American Medical Association* on December 3, 1932, immediately after the appearance of the report of the committee above referred to, they criticized the *Majority Report,* and took their stand upon the view "that more than 80 per cent of all the ailments for which people seek medical aid can be treated most cheaply and most satisfactorily by a family physician with what he can carry in a handbag."

As already indicated, this doctrine does not appear to me to stand careful scrutiny. It savors too much of the sort of deified guesswork which was inevitable half a century ago.

A further editorial on December 10, 1932, again severely criticizes the *Majority Report* and suggests that the plans of the majority are subversive of our form of government.

There is, moreover, a far greater concern than the rights of the physician to practice as his knowledge and training indicate is desirable. There is the question of Americanism versus sovietism for the American people. There is the question of the right of the American citizen to pick his own doctor and his own hospital, to pay his own bills with his own money, to be responsible to a doctor who is responsible to him.

I should find it easier to give wholehearted approval to this view if I were satisfied that the American people had available the money with which to supply themselves with the medical and hospital care here referred to, but I do not see in the proposals of the American Medical Association any method by which such an arrangement can be brought about.

A somewhat similar view was expressed by Doctor West, the secretary of the American Medical Association, when he said, on December 18, 1932:

I stand for the principle that if any new plans for providing medical service are to be put into operation, they should be controlled by the medical profession, which is the only group qualified to know what is good and what is not good. Certain plans have been put into operation by medical societies. They have found, in most instances, that to make them go they have had to resort to the same purely commercialistic practices which have been used by purely commercialistic groups that have promoted similar plans to their own communities.[3]

This view seems to endow the medical profession with more exclusive knowledge—not only of the medical, but of the social and economic problems which are involved—than there is any evidence that it possesses. That the medical profession, acting as an expert in its own field, is the best witness on medical problems no one has denied, but the broader proposition that it must be given control of the methods by which people shall be allowed to obtain medical service is a large order, and one which it will find hard to fill.

On the whole, the official position of the American Medical Association has been violently opposed to any attempt to utilize the insurance principle, as exemplified by experiments in Europe. This, of course, is entirely proper, but it has not been clear that at all times the Association has quite fairly stated the case. Their British correspondent has not always taken a judicial attitude, and the quotations which they have used have sometimes resulted in unfair inferences. Moreover, I think they have not always assisted the profession of the country in getting at the facts and in studying the problems as much as would have been desirable. At the time that the

Michigan State Medical Society was making a careful investigation of the possibilities of introducing some form of the insurance principle, under the auspices of their state organization, it apparently did not get first-class coöperation from the parent body, as the following quotation from its publication will show.

The matter was finally presented to the Executive Committee during the latter part of December. The Chairman of the Executive Committee concluded that the subject was one that concerned not only Michigan but all the other states as well. He, therefore, concluded that the best results would be obtained if the Executive Committee met in Chicago with our employees in the national organization. The purpose of such a meeting was obvious. Michigan sought advice and guidance in the solution of its problems.

To me the results of this meeting with our employees were both unsatisfactory and disturbing. Those present, in addition to the Executive Committee and Dr. Bruce, were Dr. West, Dr. Leland, Dr. Woodward, and Dr. Cary, Ex-President of the A.M.A.

The Michigan delegation placed its problem before these men and asked for specific information.

The information requested was not forthcoming and the general attitude seemed antagonistic. While Dr. West kindly explained the workings of the A.M.A., the discourse was not on the subject and failed to answer our questions. Dr. Leland appeared to be guarding 107 pages of manuscript on the subject of health insurance, but stated he was not in a position to report. Dr. Carey magnanimously offered advice that seemed to be a bit gratuitous. He said that we should thoroughly thrash out the whole subject, that we should not involve ourselves, and that Michigan should delay lest it get into trouble. In short, the advice was "Do nothing." All this, of course, gave little information and less comfort to the Michigan Executive Committee. During the discussion, Dr. Bruce asked Dr. West certain questions concerning the publications of the A.M.A., and the answers were anything but satisfactory. The representative of the A.M.A. assured the Executive Committee of the Michigan State Medical Society that they had no objection to Michigan making an independent study of European plans.[4]

Michael Davis in a recent publication suggests that the American Medical Association has not always helped the state and county societies to the extent which might have been expected.

One would naturally assume that forward movements of county medical societies and other local bodies of physicians would have been led and coordinated by their national organization, particularly as this association had endorsed the minority report which recommended just such professional initiatives. But what are the observed actions, as contrasted with the logic of words? Plan after plan proposed by local groups of physicians or by county medical societies for establishing some organized service or for utilizing the insurance principle to help people pay the costs of sickness has been checked or stifled, usually less by open attack from national headquarters than by fomenting opposition to it from certain elements in the local professional circle. In Milwaukee during 1932 a committee of the county medical society had developed a scheme of sickness insurance to be offered to the people of their community even more comprehensive than the plans now in operation on the Pacific Coast. This plan began to attract more than local attention, but as soon as it became apparent that it might be translated from paper into operation in Milwaukee, influence was exerted from the large city eighty miles away. The plan suffered a series of adroit postponements, and it now lies in limbo in a committee, which apparently cannot dismiss it because of a real local interest and apparently will not report it out because of external pressure.

Nashville was one of the cities in which I had the privilege of discussing with the county medical society a similar plan which a committee had prepared. Six months later, one of the leading physicians of the city told me it had been decided not to try to push the plan further because of requests from one of the officials of the American Medical Association. Efforts of the same kind were made to dissuade the American Hospital Association from endorsing group hospitalization as a means of helping the average man pay his hospital bills. When this proved futile and when these hospital plans began to extend into more and more communities, a series of publications from the Bureau of Medical Economics of the American Medical Association appeared, describing hospital insurance plans, mostly those of a commercial or obviously faulty nature. Where these reports deal with sound and reputably organized schemes, they confine themselves chiefly to dangers and defects, presumably with the intent of discouraging any action. One scans these publications in vain for encouragement of that "controlled experimentation" to which the Association's editorial had referred as the method of evolutionary progress. By adroit phrasing, if not by direct statement—as in a recent editorial which refers to "all sorts of hospital insurance schemes" as "mechanizations of medical practice"—the road to experimentation is always fronted with a danger signal. It is never set with a green light.[5]

On the whole, the Association has tended to take a conservative, and at times even reactionary, view. They have suggested willingness to approve controlled experimentation, but it is not evident that they have aided much in initiating or assisting such experiments.

On June 10, 1934, the American College of Surgeons published the report of its Medical Service Board which had been studying the problem during the past year. This report said:

> The Medical Service Board of the American College of Surgeons respectfully submits the following report to the Board of Regents:
>
> 1. The American College of Surgeons affirms its interest and its desire to co-operate with other agencies looking toward the provision of more adequate medical service to the whole community.
>
> 2. The College believes that it is the duty of the medical profession to assume leadership in this movement and to take control of all measures directed to this end.
>
> 3. Encouragement should be given to the trial of new methods of practice designed to meet these needs, and a careful evaluation of their success should be the duty of the medical profession before they are offered for general adoption. All such new and experimental methods of practice must be conducted strictly in accordance with the accepted code of ethics of the medical profession in order that the interests of the patient and the community may be protected.
>
> 4. The College recognizes for immediate study four groups of the population for whom more adequate medical service should be made available, as follows:
>
>   (a) The indigent.
>   (b) The uneducated and credulous members of the community.
>   (c) Those who because of limited resources are unable, unaided, to meet the costs of serious illness and hospitalization.
>   (d) Those living in remote districts where adequate medical service is not obtainable.
>
> 5. The care of indigent sick should be a direct obligation upon the community and (unless otherwise compensated by intangible benefits such as staff and teaching appointments, opportunity and experience), physicians fulfilling this public service should receive remuneration.
>
> 6. The College should work in co-operation with other medical groups in order to dispel the ignorance and credulity of the public, and to bring the people to a proper realization of the protective and curative resources of modern medicine.

7. The American College of Surgeons recognizes that the periodic prepayment plan providing for the costs of medical care of illness and injury of individuals and of families of moderate means offers a reasonable expectation of providing them with more effective methods of securing adequate medical service.

A number of different plans for the organization of such services have been proposed, although few have been in operation long enough to permit definite conclusions in regard to their success. It is to be desired that these experiments be continued. Conditions differ to such a degree in different parts of the country that a specific plan which is practicable in one place may require modification of details in other communities. The varying restrictions imposed by present insurance laws in different states further complicate the problem.

Periodic prepayment plans providing for the costs of medical service may be divided into two classes: (A) Payment for medical service; (B) payment for hospitalization.

It is suggested that plans for the payment of hospitalization alone (Class B) without provision for payment for medical service, may be considered the first project to be undertaken in the average community.

The American College of Surgeons believes that certain general principles can and should be established, the observance of which will tend to obviate known difficulties and dangers which may threaten the success of these special forms of medical service. These principles are as follows:

(a) Periodic prepayment plans for medical service should be free from the intervention of commercial intermediary organizations operating for profit. After deduction of the clerical costs of operation of the fund and such accumulation of reserve as may be advisable in the interest of the contributors or may be legally imposed, the full amount paid by the contributors should be available for medical and hospital services.

(b) In the interest of the patient, the organization of plans for the periodic payment of medical and hospital costs must be under the control of the medical profession. The medical profession must act in concert with the hospitals and such other allied services as may be involved in the individual project, together with a group of citizens representative of the whole community and of industry who are interested in the successful operation of the plan.

(c) The principle of free choice of the physician and hospital by the patient must be assured to the end that the responsibility of the individual physician to the individual patient shall always be maintained. When hospitalization is required, this choice must of necessity be limited to the physicians and surgeons who hold appointments on the staffs of the hospitals participating in the plan or to those physicians and surgeons who are acceptable to the hospital. It is further recommended that only approved hospitals be admitted to participation in such a plan.

(d) The compensation of the physician and of the hospital should be estimated with due regard to the resources available in the periodic payment fund and should be based upon the specific services rendered.

(e) The organization and operation of any plan of this type must be free from any features not in accordance with the code of ethics of the medical profession which code has been established for the protection of the patient.

(f) The medical organizations participating in such a plan must assume the responsibility for the quality of service rendered.

8. Periodic prepayment plans for medical and hospital service should eliminate many of the conditions which have brought about the development of industrial contract practice. Until such plans have been more widely established certain general principles are here formulated with a view to the elimination of the commercial features of such forms of medical service.

(a) The Minimum Standard for Industrial Medicine and Traumatic Surgery of the American College of Surgeons should be accepted.

(b) Physicians and surgeons, qualified as in paragraph 2 of the above Minimum Standard, may properly be employed on a full time or a part time basis by industrial organizations to provide medical and surgical service for their employees, as follows:

i. To provide emergency service and first aid in injury or disease, and to provide adequate medical or surgical care for industrial injuries and diseases. Medical and surgical care of the families of employees, and of employees themselves, except for emergency and industrial injuries and diseases, should be provided by the industrial physician only in remote districts where adequate medical service is not available.

ii. To provide pre-employment and periodic physical examinations.

iii. To study the hazards of the particular industry and to co-operate with other agencies in effecting such measures as may be needed for the prevention of injury and disease.

iv. To keep accurate records such as may be required by local Workmen's Compensation laws, and so complete as to serve for scientific investigation of industrial hazards with a view to their further prevention. These records are privileged communications, subject always to due process of law.

(c) The sale of a contract by an industrial organization to an individual physician or group of physicians for medical and/or hospital service for its employees encourages commercial competition and is to be condemned.

(d) Unethical practices in publicity, advertising, solicitation, and competition, either of a professional or of a financial nature, must be eliminated.

(e) The accepted code of ethics of the medical profession, which is designed to protect the best interests of the patient, should apply to industrial medical service as to all other forms of medical practice.[6]

The whole atmosphere of this report is one of careful study by qualified people, and appears to me to take a reasonable, not radical, but yet progressive attitude. The American College of Surgeons is a group whose opinion will undoubtedly be of value to the public in coming to their conclusions, and after all, these problems can be settled satisfactorily only by the joint efforts of the public and their experts.

However, the American Medical Association objects to the expression of opinion by these experts. At the meeting of the House of Delegates on June 12, 1934, the following rather astonishing resolution was adopted by the house on the recommendation of the Judicial Council.

Whereas, The American Medical Association, including 100,000 physicians, is the only democratic body representing the organized profession of this country through delegates regularly elected through county and state medical societies; and

Whereas, Other medical organizations and groups, representing selected groups of specialists, have from time to time issued pronouncements of policies in the field of medical economics and medical practice, which do not represent the views of organized medicine and which purport to guide the medical profession and the public in the administration of medical affairs; and

Whereas, The House of Delegates of the American Medical Association has repeatedly condemned the issuing of such announcements of policies, which seriously embarrass the attempts of this organization to secure adequate care for the health of the American people and to protect the ideals of the medical profession; and

Whereas, The Board of Regents of the American College of Surgeons, assembled in Chicago on Sunday, June 10, promulgated a policy including a prepayment plan for medical care, restricted to so-called "approved hospitals" to members of the staffs of such hospitals, and to physicians acceptable to such staffs; and

Whereas, This action of the Board of Regents of the American College of Surgeons has been spread to the people of the United States through the public press on the opening day of the annual session of this House of Delegates; therefore, be it

Resolved, That the House of Delegates of the American Medical Association express its condemnation of such tactics and of this apparent attempt of the Board of Regents of the American College of Surgeons to dominate and control the nature of medical practice; and be it further

Resolved, That the House of Delegates request the Board of Trustees of the American Medical Association and the Judicial Council to ask the Board of Regents of the American College of Surgeons, who are themselves members of the American Medical Association, to explain the reasons for their action and to justify the attempt by this small group within a specialistic organization to legislate for all the medical profession of this country, truly represented only by the American Medical Association.[7]

This resolution suggests that the American Medical Association is inclined to deny the right of other bodies of qualified experts to express their opinions. That they may properly disagree with opinions expressed, and may point out that they are expressed by groups of whose qualifications to form an opinion they are doubtful is beyond question. There will be much dissent, however, from the view that they are entitled to ask the American people to accept them as the only people qualified to an opinion, and insist that their opinions shall be accepted as controlling. The public is entitled, I think, to obtain information from all possible sources, and qualified experts should be encouraged, not discouraged from expressing their opinions.

Finally, I wish to draw attention to two suggestions which commonly run through the presentations of the subject as put forward by the older physicians and by organized medicine.

One proposition is that there is not, in fact, any large number of people who are really deprived of satisfactory medical care.

The other is that the problem of financing is really a question of the willingness of people to get along without certain luxuries in order that they may pay their doctors' bills.

The Los Angeles County Medical Society in discussing this problem of medical care says:

> The problem to be solved has far deeper implications than those evidenced by certain hardships worked upon a class of people who have trouble in paying their doctors' bills when they are sick. There are but a small number of persons who really lack medical care in times of distress. There are some, of course, so conscientious that they would rather suffer and court death than call a physician when they knew they could not pay what they thought his services would be worth. But their number is extremely low, as any member of the medical profession could show by exhibiting his list of accounts receivable.
>
> The problem is not really one in which a large number of people are suffering from lack of medical care, rather they are suffering from the burden, as they feel it, of paying for this care.[8]

I have already presented evidence, which seems to me pretty convincing, that there is, in fact, a very handsome number of people in this country who are actually suffering from want of medical care. I cannot take seriously the suggestion that physicians would be satisfactory witnesses upon this point, since I cannot conceive how physicians are to be aware of the amount of illness existing in patients whom they never see.

Upon the question of the actual existence of a very large group of people whose incomes are quite insufficient to cover necessary medical expenses—to say nothing of luxuries—I present in addition to the discussion of the problem in earlier pages, the following quotation from Simons and Sinai.

> . . . The first point to determine is whether there is, in the United States, any large section of the population with an income too small to meet the cost of necessary medical care.
>
> This question would never be raised among any of those familiar with the facts. That it is continuously raised, and the existence of such a class denied by representatives of the medical professions, is one of the principal counts in the indictment of economic and social ignorance brought against those professions. There is not a single competent student of the subject who does not agree that several million of the population of this country receive incomes insufficient to purchase the fundamental necessities of life. This conclusion is indorsed by employers' organizations and trade-unions, by the United States Bureau of Labor, charity workers, economists, statis-

ticians, and sociologists of every type and attitude. It is one of the very few undisputed facts in the realm of economics. Yet, its explicit or implied denial is constantly found in writings admitted to medical and dental journals.[9]

COMPULSORY HEALTH INSURANCE

There is much thoughtful opinion, based upon careful study of social and economic conditions both in this country and abroad, which supports the view that some form of compulsory health insurance will become essential, and therefore might wisely be instituted now. Such a view is stated by Foster. After discussing the field studied by the Committee on the Costs of Medical Care he says:

> It is unfortunate that the committee, having decided that some form of group payment is absolutely necessary, did not recommend compulsory health insurance; for nothing is more certain, in the whole wide range of the committee's field of study, than that voluntary health insurance will not meet the needs of those who are in greatest need. It will not reach the unorganized, low-paid workers. It will not solve the problem of satisfactory care for all the people, which is the very problem the committee set out to solve. Already most European countries have abandoned voluntary systems in favor of compulsory systems. Yet only nine members of the committee declared themselves in favor of a compulsory system.[10]

Hamilton in a separate minority report for the Committee on the Costs of Medical Care comes to the same conclusion.

> So it seems to me, that the scheme called compulsory health insurance is the very minimum which this committee should have recommended. Its irregular incidence, and the practical difficulties in the way of budgeting, make necessary some type of collective provision against sickness. Furthermore, we have not as yet found a way to assure to all workers a minimum wage or to abolish insecurity from the economic order; and, so long as income is fitful and uncertain, it cannot provide an adequate basis for the financial maintenance of medical services.[11]

Both of these gentlemen were members of the Committee on the Costs of Medical Care, and were thus in a position to study carefully the evidence submitted.

Kingsbury comes to a somewhat similar conclusion.

> European experience shows that every voluntary scheme has been a bridge to a compulsory scheme. Experience is accumulated through volun-

tary insurance, and this is very useful in the establishment of a compulsory system. Unfortunately, many of the worst abuses which develop under voluntary schemes are carried over into the compulsory stage and remain to confuse the new administration and to interfere with efficient operation. The people in the lower-income brackets, who most urgently need an insurance plan, show the greatest inertia in coming into a voluntary plan. The poor, the mass of workers, can be only partly, if at all, covered by voluntary insurance. We propose that if insurance is to cover the people whom it should cover, both in their interest and that of the community, it must be grounded on a compulsory basis.[12]

Upon one point in regard to the question of insurance there appears to be remarkable unanimity, not only among those who approve of insurance, but those who disapprove of any plan thus far put forward. This agreement, interestingly enough, concerns itself with the futility of voluntary insurance, and the certainty that any voluntary form is but a stepping-stone to compulsion. That this view is supported by a good deal of evidence must be admitted at once, but the claim appears to me too sweeping. There is a good deal of evidence in Great Britain that voluntary insurance to cover certain parts of the cost of medical care—namely, hospital care—has been undergoing a rapid and satisfactory growth. Moreover, there is some evidence to show that even though it be true that voluntary insurance will sooner or later lead to compulsion, it does not necessarily follow that for this reason it should be refused a trial. It is just possible that the use of voluntary methods of insurance may lead to important knowledge tending to show at just what level some form of compulsion must be exercised. It does not appear to me certain that the evidence of the tendency of voluntary methods to become compulsory authorizes us to condemn them out of hand. There is ample evidence that the physicians of this country, who are, as I think, facing the problems in a realistic way, are desirous of satisfying themselves that voluntary insurance will fail before they accept anybody's opinion to that effect. That voluntary methods will be crowned with complete success is, I believe, doubtful, but I am quite unwilling to admit that the evidence justifies us in proceeding at once to compulsion on the ground that nothing else will do.

One cannot have lived in this country during the last fifteen years

LAISSEZ FAIRE OR COMPULSION   239

without experiencing grave doubts as to the effect of compulsion upon the American people. Our behavior in regard to the Eighteenth Amendment cannot safely be overlooked. At the time this Amendment was passed there was, I believe, overwhelming opinion in this country in favor of temperance. Moreover, the country was proceeding slowly, irregularly, but, on the whole steadily, toward temperance. We allowed ourselves to be stampeded into imposing compulsion. We failed miserably, not only in enforcing compulsion, but in maintaining temperance. It is possible, of course, that compulsion in regard to the question of insurance might be so concealed that it was not quite recognized by the people that it affected. I doubt whether this line of procedure would succeed.

Insofar as the compulsion, to which reference is made here, takes the form of compelling individuals to make savings and contributions to funds from which medical care will be provided, I am doubtful of its success. Certain kinds of compulsion would undoubtedly succeed. For instance, if public opinion supports it, it would be entirely possible to compel the taxpayer to contribute to funds for this purpose. It would be possible to compel corporate business to contribute, within the limits which would enable them to avoid bankruptcy. Thus far, if public opinion approves, compulsion could undoubtedly go—beyond that point I am more doubtful.

My reasons for being unwilling to approve of immediate compulsory action are not theoretical. I am aware that the American people have accepted the view that education should be supported by the taxpayer. I am aware that in many fields the community has been willing to tax itself for the common good, and to proceed slowly toward the socialization of many activities which to our grandfathers would have appeared stark socialism. Part of my objection arises from my doubt as to whether we have under our political organization the atmosphere in which such experiments can satisfactorily be tried. This doubt I have already expressed in Chapter XIII. Finally, if we assume that our present form of government, with its great dependence upon public opinion, is to continue to exist, I believe it must be clearly shown that there exists a large, well-advised, and influential body of opinion which supports any plan involving the use of compulsion. At least during the period from 1914 to 1920 when the question of compulsory insurance was last actively raised, evidence was lacking to show that organized labor favored or desired it. It will be important, I think, to take this large body of opinion into account. If the opinion has changed, then the probability of success will be increased. At the present time I do not know of any evidence tending to show that the opinion of "labor" has been canvassed, or is known to be favorable. It may well be that the long view might lead to acceptance of the doctrine of compulsion, but I think there are a number of fields which must be explored before this conclusion can be accepted.

We May Develop Our Own System

As has been pointed out previously, the plans for spreading medical care more widely, which have yielded reasonable measures of success in other countries, have been universally the outcome of conditions there existing. Without repeating what has already been said, it should be remembered that the Compulsory Insurance Act in England grew directly from the already existing voluntary care under the Friendly Societies. The satisfactory plan working in Denmark is a slow development based upon long-existing conditions. It appears to me essential that we, in this country, should examine carefully the conditions, which now exist here, to see how we can build upon a foundation of our own, rather than attempt to lift institutions which have developed upon different foundations. There are, I believe, at the present time in this country fragmentary efforts which may perhaps point the way to successful further development.

THE WORKMEN'S COMPENSATION ACTS

We have already in existence a form of compulsory insurance under these acts. In most of the forty-four states which have passed these acts the burden of medical care and compensation, for injury received by the employee, has been placed directly upon the business. In the aggregate a very large number of the people are cared for under these acts. It would be a bold man who would assert that the workings of these acts have been entirely satisfactory, but it would verge upon insanity to suggest that the conditions existing since the passage of these acts are not a very important improvement over the conditions of an earlier day. No one who saw much of the difficulties of the employee under the previous system of liability laws will doubt that these acts were a step in advance.

On the other hand, if they be looked upon as a fair sample of the best that we can do in compulsory insurance, then the case for extending compulsion to ordinary illness looks to me as if it were hopeless. It seems proper to suggest that a very serious attempt be made to improve the workings of these acts. If the people of this country, as a whole, are prepared to welcome compulsory insurance for general sickness, then there should be no grave difficulty in smoothing out the constant difficulties and disagreements which have grown up under the compensation acts.

These acts were passed, as a rule, without thorough investigation, but at the present time a sufficient body of evidence exists which tends to show their weakness in practice and the measures necessary to improve their operation. Two main weaknesses of these acts are that, when passed they did not make adequate provision for medical care, and that the commissions charged with their operation are not wisely selected. Another serious difficulty grew out of the lack of appreciation by the medical profession of the implications necessarily involved, at the time of passage. There has been widespread failure in coöperation between medical organizations and the administrative bodies. Experience in other countries seems to me to point clearly to the fact that these acts should be administered by non-political appointees, that the commissions should contain one or more physicians, and that there always should be connected with these commissions an advisory board consisting wholly of physicians. I think it probable that the workings of these acts would be improved if the chairman were a physician. Satisfactory results are not to be expected unless, and until, we can separate such commissions from politics, and unless the services of trained people, who will continue to hold office over long periods of time, can be obtained.

Another grave difficulty inherent in these acts appears to me to arise out of the creation, by many of them, of the insurance carrier. Here is necessarily introduced the element of profit. I cannot bring myself to believe that the care of the health of the community is a proper subject for private profit. No examination of the history of insurance carriers, whether under these acts, or others, can fail to show that the profit motive is working here to the disadvantage of the beneficiary. It is perhaps true that the states which have set up "exclusive" state funds have not always succeeded in managing their problem better than the states in which insurance carriers do a large part of the work, but from this it does not appear to me to follow that the exclusive state fund is not, on the whole, the better general method. It may appear that self-insurance and mutual funds are an improvement over the principle of the insurance carrier, but both appear to me to violate the basic principle that the care of the sick at levels where the state feels required to intervene should not be made the subject of private profit.

Where exclusive state funds have been established, and to the extent that in the future this method becomes more common, it will be of the first importance to remove the commissions in charge of administration from political influence. This, together with the requirement of relative permanency of tenure, would certainly improve administration. It would be a step in the direction of developing permanent agencies to deal with this and similar problems. It seems probable that, at some level, further provision will have to be made, which look to contributions from taxation to provide medical service for the indigent. The establishment of relative permanency in commissions handling workmen's compensation would be an important step toward the development of similar permanent bodies in other fields of health service. Every effort should be made to remedy the defects of this type of compulsory health service before we take any further steps in that direction.

ENCOURAGEMENT OF VARIOUS PLANS FOR VOLUNTARY INSURANCE

There are many of these plans in a considerable variety of fields. All of them probably should be regarded as experimental. Most of them have failed to receive encouragement from organized medicine. On the other hand, at least some of them are experiments which, if they are given a reasonable opportunity, will, I believe, add importantly to the evidence which is now inconclusive or lacking.

Community medical service.—In various parts of the country experiments have been tried in the extension to the community of medical service, which has been built up under industrial auspices. The experiment at Roanoke Rapids was previously discussed. It is, perhaps, a favorable instance of such a development—since it has been set up in a group of Southern mill towns, where satisfactory medical service has been difficult to obtain in the past. Such experiments, as a rule, have not had the support of the medical profession, probably because they introduce into the sphere of medical competition an unpredictable quality to which objection is made, partly because it is new, and partly because it suggests the possibility that free competition may not be the best method of procedure.

It does not seem to me doubtful that these experiments have improved the offering of medical service in a number of instances. Their possibility of survival depends largely upon the attitude taken in regard to them by organized medicine. I think that they can be destroyed by adverse action. I am hopeful, however, that such action will not be taken, for the evidence appears to me to support the view that at certain stages of industrial development, and in certain parts of this country, they furnish the best available method of improving the offerings of medical service. If organized medicine would assist rather than hinder their development, if the state or county medical societies would in good faith offer their aid and assistance, not only would progress be made, but the standing of the profession at the bar of public opinion, I think, would be improved.

Private group medicine.—As already suggested, physicians organized in private groups have attempted, in various parts of the country, to widen their sphere of usefulness by offering medical care on a prepayment basis to various groups of citizens. This appears to me a desirable extension of the work now done by medical groups, particularly in the larger centers of population. Such offerings seem less applicable to the smaller communities and the regions of scattered population. In the large cities there are today very large numbers of individuals who, for one reason or another, have not attempted the difficult task of selecting for themselves a general medical adviser. They see, and I think properly, in the medical group a partial solution of their problem. It will avoid for them the task which is even more difficult than the wise selection of a general practitioner, namely, the selection of a variety of specialists. In the properly organized group both the general and the special departments are represented. It offers to these people relatively complete medical service of good grade. It simplifies for them difficult matters of choice, since they need only satisfy themselves that the group offers a good article for sale, rather than make a number of difficult choices. That offering of medical care on a prepayment basis may be undertaken by groups insufficiently equipped to do the work, is not a sound argument against the method. It is within my knowledge that such offerings by groups, which I believe to be properly equipped, have been killed by organized medicine for reasons which seem to me very unsound. In at least two instances I am aware that the members of the groups were given the choice between terminating their contract and being ostracized from organized medicine, through cancellation of their memberships in the county and state medical societies and thus, automatically, in the American Medical Association. Such action does not promote unity in the profession, does not lead to conviction that organized medicine can be trusted to take a judicial attitude on economic questions, and, among the younger group of physicians, serves largely to increase the unrest due to the quality of control exercised by their elders. Dr. Rexwald Brown states a somewhat similar view, in part as follows:

> Opposition to group practice looms large in the mind of the uniformly trained medical man. His opposition is centered about the fixed conviction that freedom of choice of physician by patient is annihilated in group practice. No individual of the opposition thinks that perhaps the manner of practice for centuries might be changed for the better.[13]

A much sounder policy for organized medicine would be that of offering to coöperate with such groups, to assist them in arranging the proper terms of what amounts to a contract, and to act in an advisory capacity in regard to the maintenance of a high level of professional service. Handled in this way, such experiments would sink or swim, chiefly on the basis of the soundness of their offering. As the situation stands, they sink or swim, largely through the whim of people whose hindsight is better than their foresight.

Voluntary insurance under the auspices of county medical societies.—This is perhaps the outstanding instance in which organized medicine has not opposed the experiments in voluntary insurance. In some states careful investigations have been made and plans set up that are based upon a reasonably thorough knowledge of somewhat similar experiments in other countries. As already indicated, none of these plans has been in operation long enough to warrant any satisfactory opinion as to their workability.

The plan recently put forward by the Michigan State Medical Society is among the most complete, and though it apparently failed to receive the blessing of the American Medical Association, its development should be watched closely, and should be assisted in every feasible way by everyone interested in the development of voluntary insurance.

That this plan will not receive the unanimous support of the physicians of Michigan is suggested by the following editorial from the Wayne County Medical Society:

The sociologists state it is inconceivable that any form of health insurance can exist without unemployment insurance. This writer must agree that to try to do this spells evasion, cowardice or stupidity. This is our major objection to the plan proposed at the state meeting. Any honest approach to a disorganized, disjointed, creaking social system will not . . . put into effect a plan that seeks to bolster up economic inequalities. . . .

For a glance at the cost of State Medicine and its satellites, let's look to Britain, a land with one-third the population and one-half the wage standard of America. Neville Chamberlain, Chancellor of the Exchequer, estimates the yearly expenditure of the British Isles, ending March, 1935, for protection, health and dole as follows:

Army	£31,418,000	($161,000,000)
Navy	£47,208,000	($244,000,000)
Health and Labor	£147,526,000	($763,000,000)

Health and Unemployment insurance cost $520,000,000 more than the cost of building and maintaining the world's biggest navy!

Let's have the sociologists (well paid by Foundations) sell health insurance and its expensive companion, unemployment insurance, to the thoughtless people (including the doctors) who will hereafter and eternally fight the exorbitant taxes necessary to maintain these bureaucracies in political-spoils America (is Britain as full of political pork as America?) until the load becomes unbearable. . . .

Verily, after Health Insurance will come the Deluge! [14]

The objections here voiced are apparently very inclusive, and appear to take their stand against the whole proposition of social insurance and particularly unemployment insurance, as a corollary to which compulsory health insurance has often developed. There is very widespread opinion in this country, at the present time, supporting the view that the stabilization of industry looking to the avoidance of periodic economic crises will require some form of unemployment insurance. This opinion is apparently shared by President Roosevelt. Wholesale opposition to such fundamental economic plans, I think, will not increase the confidence of the public in organized medicine as a sound source of economic guidance.

Hospital insurance.—By this phrase it is intended to indicate various experiments under which groups of hospitals undertake to insure people in the lower income-brackets, so that they will receive hospital service when it is required. This has already achieved some success in Great Britain. It is but in its infancy in this country. It serves to relieve the individual of a part of the burden of unexpected illness. It is not a solution of the problem of medical care for people of the class mentioned above. On the other hand, it may easily go hand-in-hand with other developments of service on a prepayment basis, and be amalgamated into a valuable whole. It is likely to be most useful in relatively large centers of population where the supply of hospital beds is, as a rule, somewhat in excess of the average need. It will be less valuable in the more isolated communities where hospital beds are less in excess, and where there are fewer hospitals who can combine to make the offering. The profession would be well-advised to lend the weight of its authority to the principle here involved. There will be a variety of obstacles, some legal, some technical, some administrative, which can be surmounted only by cooperative action.

An interesting study has been made by Walsh, who reviews the problem carefully, and after careful study. He notes the resistance of the medical profession as follows:

> The organized medical profession through its national, state and county organizations, quickly sensed the dangers of plans sponsored by agencies activated by the profit motive and has used its powerful influence against the development of all plans of this nature—good, bad, or indifferent.[15]

The American Hospital Association, I believe, is more or less committed to the plan. Organized medicine has up to now held rather aloof. If these two groups cannot agree, the plan will probably come to nothing.

INDUSTRIAL MEDICINE

It will not be necessary here to review what has already been said in regard to this field. That it is an important field is clear because it is primarily based upon the requirements of the Workmen's Compensation Acts. There is no prospect that these acts will be repealed; there is considerable evidence that they are being steadily extended to cover not only industrial accident but industrial disease.[16] The inclusion of industrial diseases closely approaches compulsory health insurance. Organized medicine has treated this field rather like a poor relative, and has consistently held the view that, even for work likely to be as technical as the management of industrial injury and industrial disease, the general practitioner is entirely competent and that freedom of choice must be demanded for the employee. A recent survey of this field made under the auspices of the American College of Surgeons lists the following qualifications for an industrial physician, whether he be on full-time, part-time, or a call basis:

1. He should be a graduate of an accredited medical school and licensed to practice in the state or province.
2. He should have at least one year's internship in an accredited hospital.
3. He should have some experience in general practice either prior or supplemental to his duties at the plant.
4. He should be qualified to determine by examination of employees their physical and mental fitness for work.
5. He should have a general knowledge of industrial relations, including employment methods, special problems relating to the employment of women and children, recreation, transportation, housing and educational facilities and methods, and employees' benefit plans.
6. He should have a knowledge of the ingredients and of the toxic or disease producing nature of all the materials and processes used in the industry and of applied preventive medicine in general.
7. He should have a knowledge of the diagnosis and treatment of occupational diseases.
8. He should have a knowledge of sanitation, of working conditions, and of accident prevention methods.

9. He should be competent in the diagnosis and treatment of all traumatic lesions which he undertakes to treat.
10. He should be versed in procedure for follow-up and rehabilitation.
11. He should have a knowledge of the compensation laws involved and of an efficient record system including statistical methods.
12. He should have an unbiased industrial viewpoint and a confidence-inspiring personality.

Criticism has been made by members of the medical profession that some of the above qualifications of an industrial physician are superfluous, and they contend that the doctor should adhere to the practice of medicine and surgery for which he was trained. A physician may come to an industrial organization skilled in medicine and surgery, and yet fail in satisfying all of the industrial requirements. The additional required qualifications make of industrial medicine a specialty. Without such interests and qualifications the general practitioner or plant physician cannot expect to serve industry adequately as a medical director or advisor.[17]

Such a list of qualifications from such a source should, I think, be taken seriously. It is in line with the opinions which have long been held by industrial physicians whose experience qualifies them to give an opinion. It has been satisfactorily shown that, under the care of men with these qualifications, accident, injury, and industrial disease stand a significantly better chance of prompt and satisfactory recovery than under the care of the average general practitioner.

Obviously, the satisfactory care of their employees is a matter of primary importance to industry, and one which will become progressively more important as industry becomes more complicated, as the number of diseases peculiar to industry increases—as it certainly will—and as the importance to the employee of maintaining his working ability becomes more evident, with advancing years. Here is needed close coöperation between organized medicine and organized industry. This can be worked out most easily in the case of large industries employing a relatively large number of men.

Unfortunately, $75\frac{1}{2}$ per cent of the total factory workers are employed in establishments having less than 1,000 employees; approximately 30 per cent are in those having less than 100 employees. It should also be noted that the injury frequency rate is highest in those plants with a small number of employees, and diminishes steadily—being lowest in those employing 1,000 or more.[18] Here obviously is an important problem. It appears that in the larger plants with relatively complete medical plant organization, the service is satisfactory, but in the plants too small to afford such an organization, the care rapidly diminishes in excellence as the number of employees gets smaller.

Attempts to solve this problem, by the establishment, in various cities, of medical groups organized to deal chiefly with industrial accident and injury, does not seem to have worked satisfactorily. It is obviously a difficult problem in which the element of commercialism will enter very easily, and one in which, by the same token, the quality of service is likely to decline. It should be possible, in any given locality, to indicate the physicians having the necessary qualifications to offer industrial service. Among these, choice should be allowed. It should be possible to so supervise and oversee their offering of medical service as to hold them to a satisfactory level. Such a result can only be obtained by self-policing by the profession to an extent which has not been undertaken as yet. This problem of government within the profession is one to which I shall have occasion to refer later. However, I do wish to indicate that industrial medicine, certainly for those types of injury and disease coming under the Workmen's Compensation Acts, has developed to a point where it should be regarded as a specialty. The profession should supervise the qualifications of this group of specialists, utilizing the same standards which they apparently are proposing to exercise in regard to the more generally recognized special fields. That the general classification and supervision of specialists are important, seems to me obvious, but in this particular specialty, medicine finds itself able, if it will, to coöperate with industry. Such coöperative efforts can be made very much more effective in the future than they have been in the past. As already indicated, I think I see evidence that industry is becoming more social-minded. Here is an opportunity for organized medicine to demonstrate that *it* is socially minded and abreast of the current problems of social economics. Neither industry nor organized medicine can succeed in this field except by coöperative methods, but by those methods, I believe, great improvement is possible.

Contract Medicine

It is extremely difficult to make any clear statement as to the position which contract medicine ought to play in long-distance planning. It has probably been at the bottom of more quarrels and disagreements than any other phase of medical practice. In and of itself, it is an unobjectionable method. On the other hand, it is commonly so closely associated with purely commercial ventures that it has been extremely difficult to maintain satisfactory professional standards. That it is a necessary method of carrying on medical practice in isolated industrial regions seems fairly clear. That it is a wise method for general use, except under such conditions, seems considerably more doubtful.

The difficulties which have led to disagreement have been from two sources: (1) the very common tendency to divert the primary intention, of providing medical care, into a profit-making operation; (2) the opportunity which it has given for a most undesirable competition between physicians and organizations of physicians, in seeking contracts.

1. Unless, and until, public opinion is willing to support the doctrine that the provision of health service is not a proper field for private profit, I see no method by which the desire for profit can avoid leading to serious difficulties. It is by no means clear to me that public opinion at the present time, or in the immediate future, will take any such view. It is, after all, one of the hazards which modern medicine must face in its attempt to reconcile professional standards to a commercialized environment. As I have previously indicated, the possibility of so doing seems to me gravely doubtful. Just so long as there is approval of the profit motive in this field, just so long will professional standards suffer and poor service be likely to result.

2. Competition for contracts under this system has been one of the points at which the greatest strain has been put upon the moral fibre of physicians. Under the fierce competition which now exists within the profession, it is not to be expected that underbidding for contracts, and slovenly work resulting from the taking of contracts

at rates which are in fact below the proper cost, will be avoided always—or even generally. I think it doubtful that the power of organized medicine to control and discipline its own members is sufficient to remedy this difficulty. I suspect that it is inherent in the present fierceness of competition, and is one of several situations which at least raise the question of the soundness of relatively free competition in this professional field.

XV

WHERE DO WE GO FROM HERE?

THE ORGANIZATION OF THE MEDICAL PROFESSION

The phrase "organized medicine" has come into common use in medical publications only in recent years. It has occurred largely because of the requirement that the profession adjust itself, if possible, to its commercial surroundings. Originally, medical organizations were for purposes of conferences on medical subjects. A study of the organization and development of the American Medical Association will show that for many years it was concerned primarily with bringing together physicians from all parts of the country, for the intercommunication of medical knowledge. Of course, for many years it has been required to act through its Judicial Council (1873) on questions involving disputes and disagreements occurring within state societies, and also through its Council on Medical Education and Hospitals (1904) on questions of educational policy. Only within recent times has there been any organized attempt to study, discuss, and act upon social and economic problems. At a very much earlier day it is probably true that physicians, as individuals, were relatively well informed on social problems—particularly in their immediate environment—and on the general economic problems of the country. As time went on, however, the necessity of devoting any spare time to study in order to keep themselves abreast of the times, has tended to render the physicians, as a whole, less familiar with these problems. As regards their provision for medical meetings and mutual interchange of ideas, there is probably no group in society which has kept itself so well abreast of the times. This, of course, does not mean that every physician is thoroughly up-to-date. It does mean that, as a body, physicians have for many years recognized the importance of making their studies and experiments available to their colleagues. This is wholly in line with the highest attributes of the profession, since it has always been one of the fundamental requirements of medical ethical standards that discoveries or possible improvements must be made available to the whole profession—not only nationally, but internationally—at the earliest possible moment. In its organization for the interchange of medical ideas, the medical profession stands preëminent. As regards its knowledge and investigation of current social and economic questions, this has not been true. Physicians, together with other groups, have been rather slow to appreciate the changes in these fields, and, perhaps inevitably, have been so concerned with the intricacies of their own occupation that they have been unable to keep themselves well informed in other fields.

The development of various forms of socialized medicine in European countries served to draw attention to the possibility that similar situations might arise here. On the whole, however, the medical organizations were slow to appreciate the importance of familiarizing themselves with these changes. One notes the establishment by the American Medical Association of the Committee on Medical Education and Hospitals in 1904, the establishment of a Bureau of Legal Medicine in 1922, but it was not until 1931 that there was organized the Bureau on Medical Economics. Somewhat more slowly, in the state and county societies committees on medical economics have been established. Too often in medical discussions during the last decade there has been evidence of a lack of knowledge of the world's experience as it concerns the problems which have developed in this country. If the physicians leading these discussions had been talking upon medical problems, they would at once have found themselves required to give a very much clearer account of the reasons for their opinion, and would have found their audiences seriously dissatisfied with the presentation of rather unsupported evidence. This difficulty, I think, has been overcome somewhat of recent years. At the present time these problems are being discussed with a better background of knowledge. That this is a field in which physicians through their organizations must be well abreast of ascertained fact and current opinion requires no demonstration.

Very closely linked with the problems of medical economics are the problems of the relation of the medical societies to the machinery set up by the state for dealing with medical conditions, chiefly under the compensation acts. If physicians are to hold their own, and exert the proper weight of their opinion on questions affecting the organization of the public health, it will be important that for this purpose they set up committees which are relatively permanent. Particularly is this true where physicians are required to deal with state commissions or other state officers, since a constant and continuous policy is of the first importance. In establishing such committees in medical organizations the tendency is to staff them with senior—and consequently busy—practitioners. These men may be able and willing to give their time, but they can rarely afford to do so over a period of years. The weakness of the position taken by organized medicine often has lain in the fact that members of these committees could give the requisite amount of time only at great sacrifice of their professional work. Consequently, a rather rapid rotation in the membership of these committees has resulted in lack of continuity, and consequent lack of established policy. Obviously, it will be difficult for these associations to find members who are both able and willing to give the necessary time. On the other hand, I am convinced that this aspect of the question is important. Particularly in dealing with such state bodies as industrial and accident commissions, the element of time is of great importance. Commonly enough, no conclusion satisfactory to the parties concerned can be reached, except after prolonged discussion, because it is often necessary for the representatives of organized medicine to conduct a considerable campaign of education in order that members of these commissions may understand what it is all about. Obviously the best results would be obtained if, under these circumstances, the conferees on both sides could be people with relative permanency in that position. I have already alluded to the great importance of having the membership of these commissions, as far as possible, removed from political influence. On the side of organized medicine, I think it almost equally important that the members of the committee, or at least some of the members, should be people who are able to devote a large amount of time, and that they should be continued in these positions as long as possible. Where membership of such committees has remained stable over a term of years, the largest amount of agreement has generally been found.

The Ability of Medical Organizations to Discipline Their Own Members

I have previously alluded to the rather scanty power which these organizations have over their own members. This power is based wholly upon the ability of the organization to deprive a physician of membership. Membership in a state medical society depends upon membership in the local or county society. This is the original body having jurisdiction over the conduct of its members. Appeal may ordinarily be taken from action by the county society to the appropriate committee of the state society. Under certain conditions the physician has a further appeal to the Judicial Council of the American Medical Association. But, when all is said and done, there is here no power to inflict a serious penalty.

Membership in a county or state society is a desirable thing, but there is ample evidence to show that it does not vitally affect a physician's practice, and there are a large number of physicians in the United States, who, for one reason or another, have held aloof. Their ability to develop and retain a satisfactory practice, has not been seriously affected. Any normal-minded physician dislikes to break with his professional brethren, and, under ordinary circumstances, will not do so. On the other hand, if, and when, he believes that there is a question of principle involved, he may break with the organization and suffer no serious penalty. I bring up this question, not because I am prepared to offer any remedy, but to point out the relative weakness of organized medicine in this country, as compared with similar organizations in Great Britain. There the final court of appeal is the General Medical Council. This Council does not consist of members of the British Medical Association. It is made up of one representative from each of the universities and colleges authorized to confer degrees and diplomas, five representatives of the government, and three members elected by direct vote of the medical practitioners of the United Kingdom. Under ordinary conditions, questions of discipline come to the General Medical Council only after they have been passed upon by the appropriate committees of the British Medical Association. The General Medical Council, however, is the ultimate court of appeal, short of the Privy Council. Since it is widely representative, it is freed from the suggestion that it might be directly controlled by so-called organized medicine. It is in practice a highly judicial body and an excellent court for the decision of difficult questions. In Great Britain, therefore, the power of the profession to rid itself of undesirable members is much more clear. On the other hand, the dangers of persecution of a colleague are minimized. The power of the General Medical Council of course rests upon the right to remove from the Register. That any such power could properly be given to a purely medical organization, I do not believe, since the danger of hasty and ill-considered action would be a real one. On the other hand, highly objectionable practices, such as fee-splitting, do not appear controllable under our present setup. Some more widely representative and more powerful judicial body would be desirable.

On Certain Doctrines Widely Accepted by the Medical Profession

THE FREE CHOICE OF PHYSICIANS

This phrase is constantly recurring in all discussions of the relation of physicians to society. Upon the point there seems to be extraordinarily general agreement among physicians. It may be noted, however, that the question is generally raised by physicians and not by patients. There are many instances in which medical service is supplied in such a way as to severely or completely curtail freedom of choice, and yet the patients appear to be satisfied. The point is important, since it is closely linked with another doctrine later to be discussed—namely, that of free competition. It is unnecessary to repeat here what has previously been said upon this point, but it seems proper to develop the subject a little further. As has previously been pointed out, real choice of physicians is probably among the most difficult choices that people are asked to make; yet it is insisted upon by the profession.

The Bureau of Medical Economics of the American Medical Association says:

Professional opinion in all lines, and not simply in the medical field, has become convinced by ages of experience that professional excellence is best tested by fair competition in a field of equally qualified competitors. To secure the best conditions for this test, professions have long excluded the incompetent by standards of admission and then insisted that further preference among those chosen depend on ability to convince patrons, by works and personality, of any individual superiority.[1]

This statement assumes that there is reasonable equality of professional attainment, an assumption which is obviously dangerous. It will be generally admitted by physicians that the size and value of a physician's practice bears a very uncertain relation to his actual professional qualifications. Some of the largest and most profitable practices with which I have been familiar have been acquired by physicians of very mediocre attainments.

Newsholme has encountered similar difficulty. He says:

Patients have little skill in assessing medical skill; and their choice of doctor may depend on the cut of his coat, on his social qualities, and sometimes, alas! on his plausibility in explaining phenomena which he has not accurately analysed.[2]

It is true that a study of the *Directory* of the American Medical Association will furnish considerable information from which certain sound inferences may be drawn as to the probable qualifications of a given physician, but, even among physicians themselves, the information there contained will provide only a modest basis for an opinion. Moreover, this *Directory*, in practice, is not available to the public, and consequently has little effect upon choice. It seems to me doubtful whether in the growing heat of the discussions concerning the best methods of providing satisfactory health service, this doctrine of freedom of choice can be maintained, without further classification of physicians.

With something of this in mind, the American Medical Association has undertaken the classification and registration of specialists.

On the other hand, there remains the very large body of general practitioners of whom there is no present classification, and whose capacities vary within wide limits. At the present time it would be quite impossible to come to any safe conclusion as to the experience, professional qualifications, and moral attributes of a given general practitioner. Roughly speaking, the function of this great and important group of physicians is to come to a diagnosis, wherever they may, to assist their patients in deciding in regard to the necessity of calling consultants, to carry out the ordinary methods of medical treatment, and to advise in the sphere of preventive medicine. On the other hand, as has been indicated previously, the general practitioner, by definition, has no limitations, and may—frequently does—undertake important special procedures, such as operations, without the necessary experience.

It is my strong impression that this situation does not exist to anything like the same extent in other countries. I can say with certainty that it does not exist to any large extent in Great Britain. There the line between the physician and the surgeon is drawn rather sharply. Surgery, except for emergency conditions, is not undertaken, except by members of the Royal College of Surgeons. It is true that the conditions which have existed in this country have made the drawing of such a line very much more difficult. In the past there have very commonly arisen, and there still arise, situations in which it may be quite impossible to obtain the service of a surgical specialist; whatever operation is required must be done by a general practitioner. This, however, is becoming progressively less necessary, and I believe that the drawing of such a line is becoming increasingly desirable and important in this country. It is highly desirable that general practitioners should be classified in some way so as to assist the patient in making a choice. It is obviously desirable that this classification be made by the profession itself. It would have to be made upon the basis of periodic examinations which would require a practitioner to show what fields he had thoroughly mastered, and in what fields he was relatively deficient.

A somewhat similar view is expressed by Brown: "The choice of physicians will be built on a system of repeated examination for physicians after graduation to determine their knowledge of the ever growing advancement in the medical sphere." [8]

A similar situation exists in regard to the choice of lawyers. Here there has been for many years a law directory known as the *Martindale-Hubbel Law Directory*. In it, lawyers are classified as to their experience, training, and standing in the community. This classification is not done by the profession. The information upon which the directory is based is obtained from all available sources by agents of the publishers of this directory. It is provided that no lawyer shall be classified until he has been at least five years in practice. Inquiries are then made of the judges in that region before whom he has tried cases. Inquiries are also made of bankers, business men, and other people in regard to their opinions of his qualifications. Finally, a list of his clients is available. By means of this directory it is possible to ascertain the relative standing and experience of a lawyer in distant parts of the country. I am told that it is much depended upon by people who are likely to require legal advice from a distance, at short notice. I do not suggest that this is a desirable method for use in the classification of practitioners of medicine. I put it forward merely as evidence of what has been done by the legal profession under somewhat similar conditions. The point upon which I wish to insist is that if organized medicine is to maintain its stand in favor of the age-old doctrine of freedom of choice on the part of the patient, it must do something to make available to patients evidence quite beyond that which can be obtained by the haphazard methods now possible.

Free Competition among Physicians

The doctrine of "freedom of competition" is implicit in many discussions in medical publications of recent years. It occurs frequently in connection with allegations of unfair competition, a phrase unfortunately suggestive of trade organizations. This "unfair competition" is alleged to be the result of the development of university health service, of university clinics, of other types of clinics, of closed hospital staffs, and last, but by no means least, of the development of group medical practice.

The "unfair competition" here mentioned is for financial gain. One hears no claim of "unfair competition" for the delivery of high-grade medical service. That the phrase has become more common of recent years is probably due to the fact that the rising cost of medical care has required the medical profession to compete for their slice of the income of a diminishing number of people. It is probably safe to say that not more than 10 per cent of the population of the United States have incomes sufficient to pay promptly for medical care, at a rate which will produce a satisfactory income for physicians. This, of course, takes into account the fact that the fees received from the patients below this 10 per cent are commonly not more than sufficient to pay the actual cost to the physician—the very large number, and sometimes large proportion, of patients whom physicians see, pay nothing under the present arrangements and are, consequently, an actual drain upon his resources. Particularly during the last few years, the proportion of the population able to pay full medical fees, especially that number able to pay the very large fees which are occasionally charged, has shrunk rapidly. That this shrinkage is not temporary seems to me probable, and I suspect that, in the days to come, the medical profession will find itself—if it continues to operate under the doctrine of "free competition"—competing more and more fiercely for the privilege of collecting fees from fewer and fewer people.

LIMITATION OF THE NUMBER OF PHYSICIANS

Now, as the outcry in regard to unfair competition has increased, so has the demand that the number of physicians be limited. The fact that there are today fewer physicians in relation to the population than at any time since 1850 suggests that numbers alone are not the cause of the present active interest in the subject. (See graph, p. 36.) Actuarial tables prepared for the Commission on Medical Education tend to show that, at the present rate of graduation, the proportion of physicians will not increase significantly for nearly a generation. The question of whether or not there are too many physicians depends entirely upon our decision as to what we propose to do about providing medical care for those who do not now receive it. It also depends upon whether a more adequate distribution of physicians is to be attained. That there is work which could be done to great advantage by all of the physicians now licensed in this country seems to me perfectly clear.[4] That they are not well employed, and that their incomes are insufficient, do not seem to me conclusive arguments for restriction of numbers. Furthermore, we are constantly asked to believe that, because medical practice is now carried on in what is alleged to be a satisfactory manner in Sweden, with a ratio of physicians to population of 1 to 2,890, this is evidence that anything of the kind would prove satisfactory here. As I have previously intimated, this view is based upon the proposition that we shall be satisfied with an amount and grade of medical care in this country which has been accepted abroad. This collides violently with my own observations, and I do not think that we have much to learn in regard to the proportion of physicians to population, from the experience of other countries. From an economic point of view, the doctrine of free competition and the doctrine of limitation of numbers are incompatible. The whole theory of competition means that it shall take place without limitation of numbers—and in fact be really free. Now, I do not myself believe in the doctrine of free competition, whether in this or in any other field, and I gravely doubt whether any such situation has ever existed. On the other hand, it seems to me that to clamor for limitations ill-behooves those who support the doctrine of free competition. They cannot have it both ways. They may either have free competition, or limitation of numbers.

If we proceed upon the theory that the number of physicians in this country is at least sufficient, and that limitation by some method ought to be undertaken, I think we should be willing to admit that this is a general and not a special doctrine. It is quite certain that if there are too many doctors, there are also too many lawyers, far too many architects, perhaps too many engineers. If limitation in one field is regarded as so important, the doctrine appears equally applicable to others. Once we adopt the theory that it is the business of the state to limit the number of persons who may engage in a given profession or trade, we are at once faced with an amount of denial of freedom of action which may well have far-reaching consequences. I hesitate to accept this doctrine, except insofar as it can be based upon the proposition that medical education, as at present conducted —at least in some schools—is gravely defective. To the extent that we can diminish the number of physicians by insisting that the schools in the lower classes shall come up to the standards of those in the higher classes, we shall in fact be insisting not upon limitation of numbers, but upon increased ability.

That the doctrine of limitation of numbers has wide support, and by people wholly competent to express an opinion could be shown by a large number of quotations. From these I select one coming from the address of the President of the American Medical Association. That he is a person qualified by education, training, and experience to express an opinion on this subject, no one familiar with the facts will deny. The following quotation will, I think, fairly show the case as he states it.

It requires no special actuarial philosophy to forecast what such a state [referring to the high proportion of physicians to population] will mean to the economic welfare of the future practitioner.

It is only natural to place the responsibility with the medical schools, in that they hold in their hands the power to control the supply of physicians for the future, but the time has arrived for the American Medical Association to take the initiative and point the way. During the coming year the Association, through the Council on Medical Education and Hospitals, will institute a resurvey of the medical schools of this country. Whether the problems of this new day in medicine will be met by a limitation in the number of existing institutions or the number of students admitted cannot be foretold, but it will require real courage and tenacity to bend the educational processes to the urgent social and economic needs of the changing order. A fine piece of educational work could well be done if we were to use only one-half of the seventy-odd medical schools in the United States.

It will be claimed that to close educational doors of any kind to ambitious youth is undemocratic and un-American; that, if a young man or woman wants to study medicine and can pass the necessary examinations, he or she should be free to do so. Yet, if I read the signs aright, the truly democratic process will be to take thought about the good of the whole, and less about the special satisfaction of the few. In one of the enlightened democracies of the old world, Sweden, this is being successfully accomplished. It will also be argued that in a democracy of forty-eight states the control of the number of physicians to be licensed is the prerogative of the individual state. A precedent has however been established by our neighbor to the north in the province of Alberta, where legislation was recently adopted that no more physicians will be registered in the province until the proportion has risen to 1 for 1,200 of population.

The present system opens the responsibilities of medical service not only to a larger number than can support themselves properly but to many who have not the basic qualifications for the study and practice of medicine.

The wise selection of fewer students can well be left to the educational faculties. It is now well recognized that the yardstick of basic qualifications is not confined to academic grades, for it is more important and fundamental that the prospective medical student have those attributes of personality characterized by an alert imaginative mind, physical and moral vitality, honesty, loyalty, resourcefulness and adaptability. He must be the kind of person who can deal effectively with sick lives as well as damaged organs or impaired physiology.

Much of the present unrest and anxious emotion about state and socialized medicine is the result of economic fear and uncertainty and in large part due to the social dangers that have developed as the result of an overcrowded and ill distributed body of doctors.[5]

It will be noted that he holds the view that the initiative for such limitation should come from the American Medical Association. That this is the group most immediately interested will be obvious, but one may properly shy a little at the doctrine that initiative for limitation of numbers should be undertaken by those who will obviously and immediately benefit by such action. That such procedure is more characteristic of trade and craft associations does not appear to disturb him, since in a previous address he said:

The responsibility to a large extent rests with the medical schools, for they hold in their hands the power to control the supply of physicians for the future. In the trades and handicrafts it has been the invariable practice sanctioned by years of tradition to limit the entry. In the medical profession similar limitations will have to be recognized, but medical standards must be maintained to assure adequate medical service to the public. . . .[6]

I confess I hesitate to adopt his view that the methods used by trade associations will be appropriate here. The doctrine appears to me to be a violation of the essence of professions in general, and the profession of medicine in particular. If now we assume that the American Medical Association is about to initiate a campaign for such limitation, it is proper to inquire along what lines they may be expected to proceed. Quite obviously, as I think, if numbers are to be limited, it must be done by the federal government and not by the individual states. It would be difficult to sanction any method by which individual states could limit their numbers and thereby terminate the free interchange of professional men which is fundamental in our political system. This does not appear to disturb Dr. Bierring, who apparently approves of the limitations already placed upon the number of physicians by the Province of Alberta in Canada.

One of the gravest difficulties which will be encountered will be to impose limitation of numbers upon tax-supported schools. There are, I believe, substantial legal difficulties which might have the effect of estopping a tax-supported institution from carrying out any drastic limitation. However this may be, such action would be extremely likely to have the effect of alienating the political support which is necessary to the survival of these institutions. My own experience in this field has led me to the opinion that attempts to limit drastically the students of such institutions are likely to have serious political repercussions. Again, it might well occur that there are certain states in the Union whose income is not sufficient to support a thoroughly satisfactory medical school. The suggestion that a state already having a medical school should abandon it would meet, I think, with public opposition. If it be agreed, as seems to me obvious, that there will be difficulty in imposing limitation of numbers upon tax-supported institutions, particularly if this action is taken on the initiative of an organization of physicians, it follows that the limitations may have to be made in the number of students graduated from the endowed schools. In many cases, such schools are among the best in this country, and will be found among the higher levels in any careful classification of schools. On the face of it, limitation in numbers in these schools would have the effect of diminishing the excellence of the product, and would therefore violate the whole theory of such limitations. No one, as far as I know, suggests that limitation should be carried out except with the maintenance of standards at least as high as those maintained by the higher of the Grade A schools. This results in a dilemma which will be difficult to solve.

Dr. Bierring very properly insists that academic grades do not satisfactorily measure the equipment of the prospective student for the practice of medicine. With his insistence upon quality of mind and soundness of character I am wholly in accord. On the other hand, my experience, and I suspect his, in the actual business of selecting a relatively small number of students from a very large list of applicants has convinced me of the great difficulty of ascertaining with any degree of accuracy the qualities of mind and of character which are so desirable. The educational authorities have not yet supplied us with any satisfactory method of discovering these qualities. At the present time, I shrewdly suspect that academic grades still form the largest basis for selection.

For these reasons it seems to me that the whole problem of limitation of numbers is one of extreme difficulty. I do not think it can be done upon sound economic premises without some alteration of the theory of free and open competition. I do not think it can properly be done upon the initiative of the beneficiaries, and I am not clear that there is any other body equipped to undertake it. If done at all, it must be done as a matter of public policy, and consequently must be approved as such. Any limitation should therefore be directed by representatives of the public, and not of the beneficiaries. Finally, it seems to me implicit in the doctrine of limitation that this limitation can be done only upon the grounds that it is of advantage to the public. That it will redound to the advantage of the remaining physicians, at least from a financial point of view, is the reason why, at the moment, it is so much desired, but if it is in the public interest, it will involve some very considerable extension of the oversight of the medical profession by representatives of the public.

Even at the present time, medical practice in this country has some of the attributes of a monopoly, at least to the extent that only those who have been licensed to practice are allowed to do so. The suggestion of sharp curtailment of numbers brings this aspect of monopoly further into relief. If it is proposed to set up a stark monopoly with limited numbers, then it seems to me essential that such a monopoly should be carefully regulated by the state, particularly in relation to its financial aspects.

It is my best guess that competition in this field, as in others, will require curtailment, at least if one interprets the phrase "competition" to mean competition for financial gain. The competition in which the medical profession appears to the best advantage is competition for excellence of work, for devotion to duty, for advancement of science, not for dollars and cents.

The matter is one of such obvious importance to the future of the country that, I think, it should be dealt with broadly and wisely. At the outset some group or commission widely representative of both the public and the profession should attempt to decide what should be the proportion between physicians and population. Of course, this will involve careful consideration of the extent to which we propose to extend medical service to those who do not now get it in a satisfactory way. Next, it appears to me that the general oversight of the practice of medicine will have to be transferred from a state to a federal basis, and some board set up—perhaps similar, in some respects, to the General Medical Council of Great Britain—that shall have the oversight of the whole question. Finally, this, or some other board, will have to oversee the workings of the monopoly which has thus been created. The supply, and sound training, of physicians must be maintained. Free competition between individual private practitioners, as we think of it today, does not seem to me workable under a controlled monopoly. It seems to me implicit that, if we are to insist upon limitation of numbers, we shall have to accept very severe curtailment of anything approaching the present private practice of medicine. If the demand for limitation of numbers is to be pushed, then some of these implications ought to be taken into consideration.

Charity Medical Service in Relation to the Income of Physicians

There seems to be no dispute in regard to the proposition that the amount of work done by the physician—and for which he receives no compensation—has on the whole tended to increase, and has increased very rapidly during the last three years. To the extent that the conditions of these recent years are highly abnormal, this increase may properly be discounted, but it remains true that a very handsome proportion of the time of many physicians is spent in caring for patients, free of charge. This is an old and inspiring ideal coming to us from the past, directly related to the fact that the profession of medicine, together with those of law and education, sprang primarily from the church. It is part and parcel of the whole ideal of service—one which the physicians will sacrifice with reluctance. On the other hand, it is with the gravest difficulty, if at all, that such a practice can be made to fit in the thoroughly commercial setting of a modern industrial world. The two things are probably to a considerable extent incompatible. This does not involve the proposition that there will be any alteration in the custom by which the physician continues to treat a patient, who may have fallen into financial difficulties, without making any charge for his services. This, after all, is merely a form of deferred payment, since he may very properly assume that the financial embarrassment of his patient is temporary, and that in times to come he will be able to meet proper charges. However, it does involve the proposition that the continued giving of professional services for the care of the indigent and the semi-indigent is an unsound economic practice. Its perpetuation involves the perpetuation of the present sliding scale of fees, which has proved a constant source of irritation. It seems to me quite clear that, for patients properly classified as indigent, and for a certain group of patients who may be only temporarily indigent—or permanently semi-indigent—their care is a proper charge against the community.

Similar views have frequently been expressed in medical publications during the last few years. It will be sufficient to quote a few bearing on this point: Heyd says: "The present day method whereby the tyranny of hospital and dispensary administration enforces free services from their attending staff is ethically wrong and economically unsound." [7]

Booth, in reporting for a special committee of the Medical Society of the State of New York, says:

Based upon the fundamentals outlined above, your Committee recommends to the Medical Society of the State of New York the following specific propositions:

Proposition Number 1

Under plans suited to the needs of the given community, and with an organization adopted and approved by the organized medical group of that community—

The worthy poor of the community shall be treated free, and no charge shall be levied against them for any medical service whatsoever. They are properly the charge of the community, and the costs of medical treatment for them should be paid for from taxation. The physician who treats them should be paid, a minimum fee fixed by the community. To have the physician, who in most instances is also a taxpayer, carry the financial burden of their care in addition to paying his share of taxes is a social injustice because it imposes a double tax on the physician.

Indigents would be entitled to treatment in the organized hospitals of the

268   WHERE DO WE GO FROM HERE?

community, or, under authorization of health departments or social service organizations, they would be entitled to treatment by physicians at their private offices or at the patient's home at special fee rates fixed for such cases. When such service is extended to this class group by voluntary hospitals, these should be paid from public funds. Indigents who are ambulatory cases and are served by the clinics and outpatient departments of voluntary hospitals also should be made a charge against public funds. The physicians who serve in the clinics and outpatient departments of the voluntary hospitals giving this service should be paid by the hospitals.[8]

These quotations fairly state an opinion widely held by the profession. That there is opinion on the other side, the following quotation from the Report of the Judicial Council of the American Medical Association will show:

During the past year, some of the basic beliefs and principles of the medical profession have been attacked and invaded more seriously and extensively than at any time before. An organized and financed campaign for a socialized system of furnishing medical care to a large proportion of the population has apparently crystallized its plans and begun its propaganda with the millions of certain foundations backing the effort. Practice of medicine by government in all the history of medicine in this country never has invaded the field of the private practitioner with his individual families as has the United States government through the Emergency Relief Administration. This is a complete and undisguised example of "state medicine." The avidity with which in general the government's offer was received can be explained only on the basis of an acute economic situation in the profession itself. The occurrence must be considered as a temporary expedient only, due to the unparalleled stress of the times, and must be discontinued as rapidly as the stress on the profession is relieved. A number of societies refused to enter into agreements whereby their members would be bound to provide services and accept compensation directly at the hands of the government. In some instances, official committees of state medical associations and county medical societies have strongly recommended to their members that they continue to provide medical service to all in need and refuse to accept compensation from the government for such services. One of the strongest holds of the profession on public approbation and support has been the age-old professional ideal of medical service to all, whether able to pay or not. That ideal is basic in our ethics. The abandonment of that ideal and the adoption of a principle of service only when paid for would be the greatest step toward socialized medicine and shortly state medicine which the medical profession could take. All our arguments as to better service to the people, freedom of choice of doctor, individual service, and maintenance of high grade medical service by highly qualified doctors would be as naught if such service were not available to a vast proportion of the people.

There is no question that medical charity is badly abused and that the past two years of public support of vast numbers of unemployed have added thousands to that number of paupers we have always with us, people who never have worked and never will, who are content to live on public charity. It conceivably may be that this number may have become so great that the burden of their medical care should be borne by the community as are their other necessities of life. Perhaps the time has come when the profession should distinguish between the temporary and the chronic indigent and demand that the community relieve the private practitioner from furnishing free care to the chronically indigent. But the temporarily indigent, those who when able paid for medical care according to their ability to pay, should still be the charge of the medical profession in their period of distress.[9]

As I have previously pointed out, this problem has never been squarely faced by the taxpayer. The general proposition will rarely be denied, but its necessary consequences in relation to taxes have not been accepted. Sooner or later this problem must be faced, and from the funds thus contributed a certain basic income can properly be assured to physicians. If various of the plans for group prepayment for medical services, now in the experimental stage, are successful, physicians will further be assured of a certain fixed income which will tend to relieve the difficulties of the sliding scale. It seems quite clear that those facts should be brought forcibly and continually to the attention of the public. I believe there is here a source of amelioration of the present financial difficulties of physicians, particularly in general practice.

However, the whole question of the maintenance in the profession of the theory of the sliding scale of fees ought to be faced. As I have already indicated, this custom among physicians—for such it is—in practice develops into a form of graduated income tax. The difficulty is that the graduation of this tax is upon no fixed scale. If the more opulent of the population are to continue to accept the view that, for a given article of medical service, they will have to pay anything from five to thirty times the average fee, then they are, I think, entitled to know—and beforehand—upon what basis this graduated income tax—and apparently its added surtax—is to be assessed. Certainly, in other fields of taxation we make loud outcry in regard to the oppressive character of taxes upon income. The sliding scale is quite as much a tax on income as is that levied by the United States. The custom has grown up which authorizes the physician to make his charges, taking into consideration the assumed income, the probable wealth, and the social position of his patient. That this is a custom, and not a law, will be clear. However, there is some evidence that the courts are beginning to question the propriety of the method, as shown by a recent decision in Texas. It is quite apparent that this is a custom which can be changed or modified as are other customs. It is conceivable that if we should decide that some classification of physicians was desirable, we might fix certain standard fees which were termed appropriate for people in certain income-brackets. That the custom does not appear logical to an economist the following quotation from a personal communication from Professor Douglass V. Brown will show:

> Isn't the sliding-scale a complete anomaly? Given,—a necessary corollary—the payment, by the community or otherwise, for work now done on a charity basis by doctors and hospitals, why should a patient's income be considered? It isn't considered in buying anything else. If the money has been "honestly" acquired, why should *the doctor* penalize the patient for having been successful? If "dishonestly" acquired, why should *the doctor* be the individual chosen to redress social wrongs? The whole thing seems utterly illogical to me. The hospital has more justification than the doctor, inasmuch as the commodity furnished is not the same in all cases.
>
> The whole thing, moreover, works very unfairly in practice. In O.P.D.'s for example, I have seen John Jones admitted because he had to keep up a heavy mortgage on his house, while Thomas Smith was refused because he had fully paid for his house; the family incomes were almost exactly the same. I have seen Pete Robinson admitted because he had eight children, and Andrew King refused because, by limiting his family to two children, he had rather hoped to get the boy to college. I have seen one person admitted because, while his income was larger by far than that of another, he "had to maintain a higher standard of living." It would be easy to multiply instances of the same sort with respect to physicians' charges.

Even granting the necessity for some distribution according to needs, I wonder if this is an intelligent way of going about it.[10]

That the custom has tended to act like a burr under the saddle of public opinion is well-known. It has been the basis of many law suits, but short of the courts, no tribunal has been set up to adjudicate such questions. It has been suggested that committees might be set up by the medical societies which would deal with these questions upon complaint of the patient. I confess this does not seem to me the wise solution, since I again hesitate to regard the group immediately interested as the best judges of the propriety of their charges. If any such committees of adjustment are to be set up, they should include an equal proportion of laymen. Such an arrangement might ease the strain. It will not solve the difficulty.

Medical Control of Plans to Distribute the Cost of Medical Care

This is another point upon which "organized medicine" seems in substantial agreement. The phrase "medical control" constantly occurs in the writings upon the subject. A fair sample of the statements is that from the *Minority Report* of the Committee on the Costs of Medical Care. They say:

> This minority group agrees that any plan for the distribution of medical costs must have the following safeguards:
> 1. It must be under the control of the medical profession. (A "Grievance Board" to settle disputes, having lay representation, is permissible and desirable.) [11]

Statements from medical bodies of a similar nature could be multiplied very largely, but except for the adding in this case of the permission to have a "Grievance Board," they are all essentially similar. This "demand" of the medical profession has arisen largely because of their dissatisfaction with the results of lay control. It is evident that in some instances the control of medical service in industry has lacked medical supervision. It is quite clear that the offering of medical service by corporations representing lay groups has introduced the profit motive, and often has been associated with poor service. Even under the Workmen's Compensation Acts there is evidence, as has already been shown, that the commissions handling these acts would benefit by more medical knowledge. The secretary of the American Medical Association believes that that body might well be given a very much broader responsibility not only for medicine, but for government. He says:

... I think that one who surveys the wreck and ruin which has well nigh overwhelmed this country for the last two years or more and who can retain a trusting confidence in big business is, to say the most for him, a supreme optimist. And I believe just enough in the common sense and, at the same time, in the idealism of the medical profession to believe that if some of its members had been at the helm we would not have been in such a terrible fix as that in which we now find ourselves. . . .[12]

Perhaps the clearest and most positive statement is one of the ten points made by the American Medical Association at its last meeting. It reads as follows: "First, All features of medical service in any method of medical practice should be under the control of the medical profession. No other body or individual is legally or educationally equipped to exercise such control." [13]

The difficulty with this demand is that it is not clear precisely what is meant by the word "control." Obviously there are three parties concerned in this business of being controlled—the patient, the physician, and the taxpayer. As far as I know, there is no important dissent from the proposition that, on questions of the technic of medical care, the qualifications of physicians, and the quality of service, the medical profession are the experts upon which the country should rely. On the other hand, any proposition to spread the cost of care will obviously involve the taxpayer, at some point, and at another point, the public in its capacity as potential patients. From the point of view of the taxpayer, the amount now expended upon medical care is large. I think it a safe assumption that it will inevitably be considerably larger. This is predicated upon the further assumption that the supply of hospital beds available for charity patients should not be allowed to fall very substantially below its present level. Up to recent times the charity contribution to the support of voluntary hospitals has been enormous. In the year 1929-30 such hospitals received, from philanthropic sources, $135,-000,000.00. In the year 1930-31 this income had fallen to $86,000,-

000.00. In the year 1931-32 it had fallen to $40,000,000.00, and the executive secretary of the American Hospital Association was authority for the assertion that it would be further reduced in 1933.[14] This means that the income of these hospitals has been reduced more than two-thirds. I do not believe that it is reasonable to expect that the sources from which these large contributions have in the past been drawn will continue to exist at anything like their present level. The whole process now referred to as "redistribution of wealth," coupled with the enormous increase in income taxes and surtaxes in the higher brackets, can mean only one thing. The large contributions from these sources to support charitable medical institutions are going to be severely curtailed. This loss must be made up from taxation.

Now it seems to me implicit in this that any arrangement which draws to any considerable extent from taxes must be in part at least controlled by the taxpayers. In the long run, "he who pays the piper, calls the tune." It does not seem to me probable that the public will be prepared to turn over to the medical profession, which, as far as I know, has made no outstanding reputation in the field of finance, the management of the enormous sums which will be involved here. It is my best guess that, if plans are inaugurated which will involve the accumulation of reserves, the public will insist upon keeping all of these questions of finance, investment, and expenditure in its own hands. I do not believe that it is going to be satisfied with moderate representation upon what the *Minority Report* graciously calls a "grievance board."

Sir Arthur Newsholme's opinion upon this question appears to me interesting. He says:

Whether the type of medico-hygienic work be chiefly official in a voluntary setting, or voluntary work in an official setting, *it is appropriate and indeed inevitable that the giving of official grants of money must carry with it a corresponding control by the representatives of the tax and ratepayers.* Voluntary associations form a parallel case. The managing committee of the association represents the donors of subscriptions, just as the local authority represents the ratepayers, and these donors or ratepayers in the final issue determine the character and extent of the work.

This principle puts out of court the claim sometimes made that the public should supply the funds for medico-hygienic work, while the medical profession or their representatives conduct it. Definitions should be required when such a contention is made. Skilled medical work cannot be controlled by laymen, but in all business arrangements the representative lay power must be supreme. The medical staff and medical committees cannot be more than consultative, although, as is universally the case, their advice in medical details, subject to non-medical financial control, is always final. It is only by frank recognition of the fact that *medical arrangements in all matters which are not strictly and technically medical must conform to the business arrangements made by the financially responsible representatives of the public that smooth progress is possible.* . . .[15]

But there is another aspect of lay interest in these problems. It is of the first importance that any plans in which the medical profession is profoundly involved should have a handsome lay representation in order to avoid the large probability that the medical group will get out of touch with its public. As a matter of fact, I think there is some evidence to show that the medical profession is less well in touch with its public than it was some years ago.

On this point the opinion of Dr. Chesley in his *Presidential Address* to the New Hampshire Medical Society seems to me interesting and pertinent:

. . . The tendency between physicians and medical societies, toward the public, is being clearly reflected in the growing tendency to the establishment of an entirely new basis of public and professional relations, on the part of the medical profession. While the scientific importance will always be primary in the functions of our medical societies, yet the life of the world has become so changed by the accomplishments of medicine itself, and the activities of the physician so greatly modified by developments of social, economic and political character, that medical organization must recognize the importance of these changed conditions. There is a feeling, among even an intelligent part of our people, that our attitude toward these matters is negative, and that the credit for making practical use of medical advance belongs in great measure to social workers, philanthropists and public-spirited laymen.

The practice of medicine formerly was a phase which was independent of, and but little influenced by, other phases of medicine. But through our changed social conditions it has in its practical application become secondary to, and more or less dependent upon, those other phases with which the public is becoming familiar. Organized medicine today is not called upon to defend itself in a scientific way, because medicine as a science has beyond all doubt proved itself to all except the severest of its critics.

Now in meeting the demands of science, medical organization has been accomplished to the extent that its function has been adequate, but in so doing it is becoming more apparent that it has failed in proper recognition of the problem of social medicine and as a consequence, the profession is suffering from the folly of its own neglect. . . .

The physician's whole training and environment have been such that his chief concern rests with diagnosis and treatment; and the act of dispensing these services becomes one of scientific aspect, but due to the fact that he expects, and occasionally receives, a reward for his services, such an act has an economic value as well. So it is evident that the practice of medicine is economic as well as scientific. The individualism and independence which exist in the private practice of medicine concentrate one's mind on his own small environment and cause him to forget or neglect its social aspect. Scientific medicine seems to have engrossed us to such an extent that we seem to believe that with this armament alone we will always be able to carry on the practice of medicine to the exclusion of all other fundamental agencies which we must admit have become of such paramount importance not only in medicine but in other professions and trades as well. It seems to me that the individual who centers his interest alone on the scientific side of medicine today, is ignoring the demands which an economic world is making on his profession and shifting the responsibility in this direction to others.

The public has been quick to recognize our failure in dealing with social and economic problems and as a result has taken the opportunity to set up lay standards of medical control in an ever-increasing expansion. . . .

The public is interested today not so much in the science of medicine as such, but in the practical application of this science. There is no question in my mind but that today the relation between the medical profession and the public is undergoing a marked change. The public is educated to what it wants. It gets from the newspapers and the radio what it expects to receive from the medical profession and it is ready to demand it, for the medical profession exists for the public and public opinion must furnish the final solution.[16]

I gather that some such idea was in the mind of Dr. Haggard when he said in an article published in the *New England Journal of Medicine* in March, 1934:

Let us analyze a little more closely what has actually been going on to develop the gap which lies between the old family doctor and the modern general practitioner. See wherein the latter has failed to carry on the tradition of public health, the tradition that he was the supreme mediator between man and his environment. And when we have completed our analysis, we shall find simply this: the public has not changed but the physician has. In becoming a modern scientist he has become less socially-minded, and, although vastly better equipped technically to do so, is less able to carry out his true function in public health work, and he desires less to do so.[17]

It is my own opinion that any board set up to manage or oversee any of these plans involving taxation should have lay representation of certainly not less than one-half. I am inclined to go further and to suggest that in the establishment of voluntary plans under which prepayment for medical service would be made, the management of such plans should have handsome lay representation.

Finally, my own experience has led me to the conclusion that, even in what is known as private group practice, the introduction of a number of laymen into the governing boards has introduced an element of stability and strongly tended to keep them in touch with average public opinion. For these reasons it seems to me unwise for organized medicine to "demand" control. I do not think they could exercise it wisely if they had it, and it seems to me that wherever the taxpayer and the public are involved, it is quite certain to be refused. The weakness of many organizations for group practice of medicine in other countries and also in this country has not lain in the fact that they were not controlled by physicians, but that the profession was not properly or even reasonably represented. It has not been my experience that the layman is unwilling to listen to the advice of physicians on technical questions. On the whole, I think he has often been too willing to listen and has tended, on some occasions at least, to swallow—hook, bait, and sinker—quite unproved and ill-considered plans. Full representation for the experts of the profession is essential. Control by physicians does not seem to me in the public interest.

Public Health Development

At the risk of repetition, I am inclined to summarize my views upon this point. This is one of the few fields of special medicine in which there is a shortage of well-trained personnel. There are not enough experts on public health questions. There are nothing like enough public health nurses to carry on work in this field as it ought to be done. It all comes down to two questions—insecurity of tenure, and lack of financial support. Until public health officers have the sort of security that they, as a rule, have in other countries—and certainly have in Great Britain—a security which carries with it a reasonable stipend, permanency of appointment, and a pension, one cannot expect to attract a large number of capable men to this field.

If the phrase "public health nursing" be held to cover the allied fields of community nursing and special nursing in the districts of large cities, then it is beyond question that the public would benefit by a very great increase of the personnel. It is probably true that at the present time the special training which this work requires has not been sufficiently given. The present grossly overcrowded condition of the nursing field is demanding relief. Here is a broad outlet, awaiting only proper financing. The possible increase of health service, as delivered by public health nurses to the indigent and to persons in the lower income-brackets is enormous. Here is work which now is not being done. It is not work which should be done by physicians. It is work which should be done by nurses with proper background and training. It is, in fact, a large untilled field.

Close to, and properly allied with, this field is the development of school health nursing and school hygiene. These developments, particularly in the case of the appointment of school physicians, have in this country been frequently opposed by the medical profession. As compared with the situation in Great Britain we are far in the rear. It has frequently been said by public health authorities—and I believe it to be true—that the development of school hygiene under the guidance of school physicians and under the immediate supervision of school nurses will develop a considerable field of private practice which now does not exist. The profession has opposed such a development on the ground that it was likely to deprive them of patients.

The observation of Sir Arthur Newsholme is of interest.

School medical inspection in some American visits I have found to be strongly resented by private medical practitioners. If "the children of their patients" are to be medically examined, then these doctors contend that they must be employed to undertake it. This impracticable and unreasonable attitude still persists to some extent; but in most countries there is frank acceptance of the value of medical inspections by special school medical officers; and there is even an increasing appreciation of the fact that the discovery of ailments in scholars has led to increased medical work for the family doctor.

This "feeding" of the private practitioner with work is an actual fact, although much more of the medical work found necessary in school medical inspection is work which in the past has not been undertaken by most general practitioners, for it needs specialist skill. This applies especially to the correction of eye defects and to the satisfactory treatment of diseased tonsils and adenoids and of deformities in children.[18]

As a matter of fact, the development of school hygiene is but part and parcel of the development of a sound child health program. Even a sturdy optimist at times may doubt whether all of the medical care which we furnish to disabled adults is worth what it costs. However, there will be no serious disagreement with the proposition that if money is to be spent in watching over the health and remedying the difficulties of the population, it can be spent to best advantage on the children. The adult may well be permanently handicapped, and it may never be possible to "make him pay dividends," but the probability of dividends from healthy children is enormous. They, at least, have not been responsible for any medical condition in which they find themselves; we owe it to them to provide them with the best outfit with which to face the world, which is likely for them to be more complex than it has been for us. These developments are an integral part of the general public health program, and should be actively assisted, not only by the medical profession, but by the public.

More Complete Use of Present Medical Personnel

By way of elaborating what I have already said in various places, I wish to break a lance for the proposition that we have at our disposal in this country a medical personnel which is capable of delivering medical service quite superior to that which is to be found elsewhere. I entirely believe that under favorable conditions this personnel does today deliver a better article of medical care than is to be found anywhere else in the world. The tragedy of the situation is that while we have, on every showing, ample personnel, we are not using it. Our medical education has on the whole undergone very important improvement in the last thirty years. The younger generation of physicians will compare favorably with their contemporaries in other countries, but we have not in the past—and we are not today —using them to their full capacity. Already it has been clearly shown that one of the difficulties concerns itself with faulty distribution. These well-trained young physicians will not—and I think should not—undertake the practice of individual medicine in isolated communities where, at best, they may earn a scant living, and probably will be compelled, if they act as individuals, to offer an article of health service which they know to be shoddy. On the other hand, I quite believe that these communities would be better off with a physician, but they must be assured that this physician has at his command the capacity to offer full service. That he cannot have it in his own person is, I think, certain. He must be linked, therefore, with some medical organization upon which he can call for expert assistance and for laboratory service—whether routine or special. I have long believed that medical groups could, so to speak, farm out younger men in these communities much as our great national baseball teams farm out their recruits. With the present development of transportation, and by the use of the telephone, these youngsters could have always at their elbows the necessary general and special advice which their patients might need. A period of service of this kind in what might be called the "bush league" would give them an insight into human nature difficult to obtain in larger centers of population. They should be attached to a medical organization which, as time went on, would draw them to the center, and further develop them as the general medical advisers of the organization. I am aware that such plans have been frowned upon from the seats of the mighty, and it is not clear that such arrangements could be made financially profitable. But, I suspect that many of these communities would be very willing to guarantee a minimum income, which has already been done in certain provinces of Canada. If these men are to be left permanently in such positions, they will, I think, lose their power, and fail to deliver the best article available. But, if they be part of a larger organization, which will as time goes on move them from one post to another, a first-class article of medical service can be offered. I am aware that such a suggestion will be met with the statement that the moving of these men from their location will deprive them of the long time view of their patients so characteristic of the family physician of the earlier day. I do not doubt that this is true. On the other hand, I suggest that the linking of these men with larger medical organizations would be in the interests of a higher grade of medicine, and that this will compensate for the loss of the long familiarity which is, I think, in many cases an illusion. On no other basis does it seem to me possible to keep physicians permanently in isolated communities; yet, I believe these communities ought to have physicians.

This is but a modification of the practice now existing under the Highlands and Islands Act in Scotland. A further development of this practice, which I have recently observed on the ground, consisted in placing well-trained young surgeons, definitely under contract to the government for a period of years, at certain strategic points in the thinly settled portions of Scotland. To these strategic points are sent, from the scattered hamlets, all the cases requiring surgical care. Here, these young surgeons obtained first-class experience from which they are equipped to profit. During the period of their contract they are assured a satisfactory income. This appeared to me to be an eminently satisfactory method of combining increasing surgical opportunities for young well-trained specialists, at the same time assuring, to the thinly settled districts, good service removed from the dangers and temptations of the fee-for-service and the sliding scale of private practice.

It would perhaps be desirable in the interest of clearness to summarize somewhat the suggestions offered in this chapter and point out their bearing upon the whole problem. I have been concerned here to set forth certain social, economic, and financial adjustments which it seems to me organized medicine may wisely entertain in order that it may be in a sounder position to play its part in whatever future changes appear necessary and wise.

I have tried to point out that in the past the chief concern of the medical profession, through its organizations, has been with the advancement and diffusion of medical knowledge. More recently it has become apparent that physicians as a group have an important part to play in adjusting medical service to present needs. I have suggested that for this purpose definite types of organization should be set up within the profession which will enable it to deal with other representatives of the public in a more effective way. It seems to me wise that the profession should select capable members who are in a position to devote time and attention to social and economic problems, and to represent the profession in various discussions. The more continuous the efforts of these people can be, the better are likely to be the results.

I have pointed out and reinforced my view that the present arrangements by which organized medicine can discipline its members are not entirely satisfactory from the point of view of the Public Interest. It seems to me important that the rights of the public in having at its disposal physicians of skill, knowledge, and integrity should be scrupulously guarded. I am not clear that the present arrangements by which medical organizations seek to discipline their members are the best that can be set up. As I have seen the workings of the General Medical Council in Great Britain, which represents not the British Medical Association, but the educational, registering, political, and professional interests, it seems to me safer and more democratic. It is important to avoid prejudice, which is always likely to develop in a purely professional organization. It is essential that the effects of disciplinary measures upon the Public Interest should be reasonably safeguarded. It would, I think, be wise to entertain the possibility of setting up, for the management of such problems, some body constituted to resemble the General

Medical Council of Great Britain. This might act as a supreme court, thereby producing much greater uniformity of treatment and more certain consideration of the broad social aspects of these problems.

My discussion of the doctrines of the free choice of physicians, the maintenance of free, or reasonably free, competition between physicians, and of the knotty question of the limitation of numbers of physicians is intended to reflect my view that these are economic problems which require further consideration of the extent to which they may involve the Public Interest. What, if any, modifications of these doctrines may become necessary will depend upon what plans may be under consideration, looking to modifications of our present offering of medical care. For instance, if we do not propose to make any essential alteration of our present offering, then I should agree that the number of physicians was too large, though I should still be in doubt as to the best method of limitation. The doctrine of freedom of choice seems to me quite lacking in an economic basis unless and until the medical profession is prepared to classify its members quite accurately and in such a way as to make the possibility of selection by prospective patients an intellectual process and not largely guesswork. Finally, I am doubtful whether even the present amount of free and open competition is in line with the present tendency to restrict competition in the interests of more coöperative living.

My above-expressed opinion to the effect that physicians should be *paid* for their care of indigent and semi-indigent patients is based upon my conviction that improvement in the probable income of physicians can be best obtained by providing them with more or less reliable sources of income coming from the state, from contributions of groups that have undertaken collective prepayment methods, and possibly from arrangements to be set up under the Workmen's Compensation Acts. It seems to me desirable that a more or less definite portion of many physicians' incomes should be based upon contributions from these sources which are relatively fixed. This will allow the physician to make some calculation as to the amount of his income other than that which he may expect to receive from private practice.

To conclude, I suggest that there is a clear case for extension of work now done under the public health organizations, and that by associating younger men with already organized medical groups, the use of this valuable and not-sufficiently-employed part of the medical personnel may be increased.

NOTES

I. Medical Practice in 1890 and in 1930

1. Alfred Whitehead, Introduction to Wallace B. Donham, Business Adrift, New York, Whittlesey House, McGraw-Hill, 1931.

II. Modern Medical Diagnosis and Its Requirements

1. Commission on Medical Education, Final Report, Printed by the Commission, New York, 1932, Appendix, Table 63.

III. Our Medical Needs

1. Commission on Medical Education, *op. cit.*, Appendix, Table 60.
2. The information upon which the chart is based will be found on p. 37.
3. Lewis Mayers and Leonard V. Harrison, The Distribution of Physicians in the United States, New York, General Medical Board, 1924, p. 159, Table 1.
4. Commission on Medical Education, *op. cit.*, p. 104.
5. Mayers and Harrison, *op. cit.*, p. 45.
6. Commission on Medical Education, *op. cit.*, p. 105.
7. Mayers and Harrison, *op. cit.*, p. 167, Table 7.
8. Commission on Medical Education, *op. cit.*, p. 110.
9. Commission on Medical Education, *op. cit.*, p. 110.
10. Commission on Medical Education, *op. cit.*, Appendix, Table 104.
11. Commission on Medical Education, *op. cit.*, Appendix, Table 104.
12. Commission on Medical Education, *op. cit.*, Appendix, Table 104.
13. In 1933 the number rose to 77 by the addition of a new school in Louisiana.
14. Commission on Medical Education, *op. cit.*, Appendix, Table 104.
15. Journal of the American Medical Association, Medical Licensure Statistics for 1931, April 23, 1932, pp. 1465-67.
16. Commission on Medical Education, *op. cit.*, Appendix, Table 92.
17. Journal of the American Medical Association, Hospital Service in the United States, June 11, 1932, p. 2063.
18. Commission on Medical Education, *op. cit.*, p. 53, and Appendix, Table 5.
19. Journal of the American Medical Association, Hospital Service in the United States, June 11, 1932, p. 2063.
20. Journal of the American Medical Association, *op. cit.*, p. 2065.

21. Journal of the American Medical Association, *op. cit.*, p. 2063-77; and Commission on Medical Education, *op. cit.*, p. 54.
22. Commission on Medical Education, *op. cit.*, p. 54.
23. Commission on Medical Education, *op. cit.*, Appendix, Table 14.
24. Commission on Medical Education, *op. cit.*, Appendix, Table 14; and Journal of the American Medical Association, *op. cit.*, p. 2074.
25. Journal of the American Medical Association, *op. cit.*, p. 2073.
26. May Ayres Burgess, Nurses, Patients, and Pocketbooks. Report of a Study of the Economics of Nursing, Conducted by the Committee on the Grading of Nursing Schools, New York, 1928.

IV. THE GENERAL PRACTICE OF MEDICINE

1. Commission on Medical Education, *op. cit.*, p. 153-56.
2. Commission on Medical Education, *op. cit.*, p. 156-57.
3. During 1934 the American Medical Association has completed arrangements for the setting up of examining boards for the various specialties.
4. H. G. Weiskotten, Tendencies in Medical Practice, Journal of the Association of American Medical Colleges, March, 1932, p. 72.
5. *Ibid.*, p. 75.
6. Walton H. Hamilton, Statement, Medical Care for the American People, Final Report of the Committee on the Costs of Medical Care, Chicago, University of Chicago Press, 1932, p. 193-94.
7. Nathan Sinai and Alden B. Mills, A Study of Physicians and Dentists in Detroit, Publication No. 10 of the Committee on the Costs of Medical Care, Chicago, University of Chicago Press, 1929.

V. SPECIALISTS AND GROUP MEDICINE

1. C. Rufus Rorem, Private Group Clinics, the Administrative and Economic Aspects of Group Medical Practice, as Represented in the Policies and Procedures of 55 Private Associations of Medical Practitioners, Publication No. 8 of the Committee on the Costs of Medical Care, Chicago, University of Chicago Press, 1931.
2. Sir Arthur Newsholme, Medicine and the State, Baltimore, Williams and Wilkins Company, 1932, pp. 42 and 78.
3. Committee on the Costs of Medical Care, Medical Care for the American People, Minority Report Number One, Chicago, University of Chicago Press, 1932, p. 159.
4. Rexwald Brown, The Place of Group Practice in the Development of Medicine and Hospitalization of the Future, Western Hospital Review, July, 1934.
5. Sir Arthur Newsholme, International Studies, Prevention and Treatment of Disease, Vol. II, Baltimore, Williams and Wilkins Company, 1931, p. 98.

VI. Group Health Services

1. University of Michigan Bulletin, Health Service in American Colleges and Universities, Division of Hygiene and Public Health, September 11, 1926, p. 14.
2. Don M. Griswold and Hazel I. Spicer, University Student Health Services, a Study of Organization, Services Rendered, and Costs in Cornell University, Yale University, the University of Michigan, the University of Minnesota, the University of California, and Oregon State Agricultural College, Publication No. 19 of the Committee on the Costs of Medical Care, Chicago, University of Chicago Press, 1932.
3. D. B. Lowe, Industrial Health Digest, 1:2, December, 1931.
4. Niles Carpenter, Medical Care for 15,000 Workers and Their Families, a Survey of the Endicott Johnson Workers Medical Service, 1928, Publication No. 5 of the Committee on the Costs of Medical Care, Chicago, University of Chicago Press, 1930.
5. Louis S. Reed, The Medical Service of the Homestake Mining Company, a Survey of a Community Medical Service Operated Under Industrial Auspices, Publication No. 18 of the Committee on the Costs of Medical Care, Chicago, University of Chicago Press, 1932.
6. Sir Arthur Newsholme, International Studies, Prevention and Treatment of Disease, Vol. III, Baltimore, Williams and Wilkins Company, 1931, p. 336-51.
7. I. S. Falk, D. M. Griswold, and Hazel I. Spicer, A Community Medical Service Organized Under Industrial Auspices in Roanoke Rapids, North Carolina, Publication No. 20 of the Committee on the Costs of Medical Care, Chicago, University of Chicago Press, 1932.
8. I. S. Falk, Organized Medical Service at Fort Benning, Georgia, Publication No. 21 of the Committee on the Costs of Medical Care, Chicago, University of Chicago Press, 1932.
9. *Ibid.*

VII. The Workmen's Compensation Acts

1. The Bureau of Medical Economics of the American Medical Association, Medical Relations Under Workmen's Compensation, 1933, p. 62.
2. *Ibid.*, p. 62.
3. *Ibid.*, p. 58.
4. *Ibid.*, p. 58-59.
5. Revue Internationale de Médicine Professionelle et Sociale, November, 1928, pp. 67-70.
6. Connecticut Workmen's Compensation Digest, Memo. of Commissioner in Jennie Riddell v. C. Fox & Co., Ætna Life Insurance Company, Nov. 24, 1928, Vol. V., pp. 446-47.

7. Bureau of Medical Economics, *op. cit.*, p. 97.
8. R. G. Leland, Contract Practice, Journal of the American Medical Association, March 5, 1932, pp. 808-15.
9. Pierce Williams, The Purchase of Medical Care Through Fixed Periodic Payment, No. 20, New York, National Bureau of Economic Research, 1932.

VIII. THE INCOME OF PHYSICIANS

1. Maurice Leven, The Income of Physicians, an Economic and Statistical Analysis, Publication No. 24 of the Committee on the Costs of Medical Care, Chicago, University of Chicago Press, 1932, p. 21.
2. *Ibid.*, p. 20, Table 1.
3. *Ibid.*, p. 35, Table 2.
4. *Ibid.*, p. 54.
5. *Ibid.*, p. 69.
6. *Ibid.*, p. 71, Table 6.
7. *Ibid.*, p. 46.
8. *Ibid.*, p. 7
9. *Ibid.*, p. 20, Table 1.
10. *Ibid*, p. 20, Table 1.

IX. THE ABILITY TO PAY FOR ILLNESS

1. Louis S. Reed, The Ability to Pay for Medical Care, Publication No. 25 of the Committee on the Costs of Medical Care, Chicago, University of Chicago Press, 1933, p. 7.
2. Commission on Medical Education, *op. cit.*, Appendix, Table 16.
3. *Ibid.*, p. 16.
4. *Ibid.*, p. 39.
5. Louis S. Reed, The Ability to Pay for Medical Care, *op. cit.*, Table 1, p. 4.
6. Louis S. Reed, The Ability to Pay for Medical Care, *op. cit.*, Table 2, p. 5.
7. I. S. Falk, Margaret C. Klem, and Nathan Sinai, The Incidence of Illness and the Receipt and Costs of Medical Care Among Representative Families, Publication No. 26 of the Committee on the Costs of Medical Care, Chicago, University of Chicago Press, 1933, p. 14.
8. *Ibid.*, Table 2, p. 15.
9. Michael M. Davis, Paying Your Sickness Bills, Chicago, University of Chicago Press, 1931, Table 5, p. 54.
10. Falk, Klem, and Sinai, *op. cit.*, Table 2.
11. Michael M. Davis, *op. cit.*, p. 17.
12. *Ibid.*, p. 18.

X. Health Insurance in Continental Europe

1. Commission on Medical Education, Supplement to Final Report, Medical Education and Related Problems in Europe, Printed by the Commission, 1930, p. 195.
2. Sir Arthur Newsholme, International Studies, Prevention and Treatment of Disease, Vol. I, Baltimore, Williams and Wilkins Company, 1931, p. 22.
3. *Ibid.*, p. 24.
4. *Ibid.*, p. 48.
5. *Ibid.*, p. 58.
6. *Ibid.*, p. 60.
7. *Ibid.*, pp. 73-74.
8. Commission on Medical Education, Supplement to Final Report, *op. cit.*, p. 142.
9. *Ibid.*, p. 144.
10. Sir Arthur Newsholme, *op. cit.*, pp. 80-81.
11. Commission on Medical Education, Supplement to Final Report, *op. cit.*, p. 136.
12. *Ibid.*, p. 136.
13. Sir Arthur Newsholme, *op. cit.*, p. 159.
14. Commission on Medical Education, Supplement to Final Report, *op. cit.*, p. 136.
15. Sir Arthur Newsholme, *op. cit.*, p. 139.
16. Commission on Medical Education, Supplement to Final Report, *op. cit.*, p. 137.
17. Sir Arthur Newsholme, *op. cit.*, p. 140.
18. Commission on Medical Education, Supplement to Final Report, *op. cit.*, p. 187.
19. Sir Arthur Newsholme, *op. cit.*, p. 162.
20. Commission on Medical Education, Supplement to Final Report, *op. cit.*, p. 137.
21. A. M. Simons and Nathan Sinai, The Way of Health Insurance, Chicago, University of Chicago Press, 1932, p. 85.
22. Sir Arthur Newsholme, *op. cit.*, p. 162.
23. E. Liek, Die Schaden der sozialen Versicherung und Wege zur Besserung, München, J. F. Schmann Verlag, 1928.
24. Goldman and Grotjahn, Compulsory Sickness Insurance, and, Benefits of the German Sickness Insurance System, International Labour Office of the League of Nations, 1928.

XI. Health Insurance in the British Isles

1. Sir Arthur Newsholme, International Studies, Prevention and Treatment of Disease, Vol. III, Baltimore, Williams and Wilkins Company, 1931, p. 37.

XII. Medical Needs in the United States

1. White House Conference on Child Health and Protection, Committee on Public Health Organization, Public Health Organization, New York, The Century Company, 1932.
2. Roger I. Lee and L. W. Jones, The Fundamentals of Good Medical Care, an Outline of the Fundamentals of Good Medical Care and an Estimate of the Service Required to Supply the Medical Needs of the United States, Publication No. 22 of the Committee on the Costs of Medical Care, Chicago, University of Chicago Press, 1932.

XIII. Some Suggested Methods of Improvement

1. W. T. Foster, Dollars, Doctors, and Disease, Atlantic Monthly, January, 1933; and Walton H. Hamilton, Statement, Medical Care for the American People, Final Report of the Committee on the Costs of Medical Care, Chicago, University of Chicago Press, 1932.
2. J. M. Robb, What Shall Be the Attitude of the Physician Toward Insurance Plans? Bulletin of the American Medical Association, January, 1933; and E. H. Ochsner, Social Insurance, Minnesota Medicine, June, 1932.
3. I am aware that it is doubtful whether the sort of provision which is here suggested is properly called insurance. The question ultimately turns upon a definition of that word, and here I find that the experts are in wide disagreement. I allow the phrase to stand, though probably the word "prepayment" would be more accurate.
4. Richard E. Scammon, What Is Guild Medicine? Minnesota Medicine, March, 1933.
5. Evans Clark, How to Budget Health, New York, Harper Brothers, 1933.

XIV. Laissez Faire or Compulsion

1. Wingate M. Johnson, Medicine and the Middle Class, Atlantic Monthly, March, 1931.
2. Oran A. Moser, The Family Doctor, New England Journal of Medicine, May 24, 1934.
3. Olin West, The Minority Report of the Committee on the Costs of Medical Care, Minnesota Medicine, March, 1933.
4. Michigan State Medical Society, Official Proceedings, Supplement to Journal of the Michigan State Medical Society, May, 1934.

5. Michael M. Davis, Change Comes to the Doctor, Survey-Graphic, April, 1934, p. 164.
6. Report of the Medical Service Board, American College of Surgeons, Surgery, Gynecology, and Obstetrics, July, 1934, pp. 129-31.
7. Report of the Judicial Council of the American Medical Association, Journal of the American Medical Association, June 30, 1934, p. 2195.
8. This Problem of Medical Care, American Medical Association Bulletin, May, 1934, p. 82.
9. A. M. Simons and Nathan Sinai, The Way of Health Insurance, Chicago, University of Chicago Press, 1932, p. 167.
10. William T. Foster, Dollars, Doctors, and Disease, Atlantic Monthly, January, 1933.
11. Walton H. Hamilton, Statement, Medical Care for the American People, Final Report of the Committee on the Costs of Medical Care, Chicago, University of Chicago Press, 1932, p. 196.
12. John A. Kingsbury, Mutualizing Medical Costs. Survey-Graphic, June, 1934, p. 285.
13. Rexwald Brown, The Place of Group Practice in the Development of Medicine and Hospitalization of the Future, Western Hospital Review, July, 1934.
14. Editorial, Detroit Objects, Minnesota Medicine, July, 1934, p. 422.
15. William H. Walsh, The Essential Principles of the Group Purchase of Hospital Service, Bulletin of the American College of Surgeons, December, 1933, p. 22.
16. Twelve states have already acted to include industrial disease.
17. M. N. Newquist, Medical and Surgical Service in Industry and Workmen's Compensation Laws, Bulletin of the American College of Surgeons, March, 1934, pp. 7-8.
18. *Ibid.*, pp. 2-3.

XV. WHERE DO WE GO FROM HERE?

1. Medical Relations Under Workmen's Compensation, Bureau of Medical Economics, American Medical Association, 1933, p. 66.
2. Sir Arthur Newsholme, Medicine and the State, Baltimore, Williams and Wilkins Company, 1932, p. 245.
3. Rexwald Brown, The Place of Group Practice in the Development of Medicine and Hospitalization of the Future, Western Hospital Review, July, 1934.
4. As far as I know, the only serious attempt to estimate the number of physicians who could profitably be used is that of Lee and Jones. My own view is that the consultant and laboratory service which they provide is insufficient. However, their study appears to show that there is grave doubt about the oversupply of physicians. (Roger I.

Lee and L. W. Jones, The Fundamentals of Good Medical Care, an Outline of the Fundamentals of Good Medical Care and an Estimate of the Service Required to Supply the Medical Needs of the United States, Publication No. 22 of the Committee on the Costs of Medical Care, Chicago, University of Chicago Press, 1932.)
5. Walter L. Bierring, The Family Doctor and the Changing Order, Journal of the American Medical Association, June 16, 1934.
6. Walter L. Bierring, Social Dangers of an Oversupply of Physicians, American Medical Association Bulletin, February, 1934.
7. C. G. Heyd, The Medical Society of the State of New York: Our Responsibilities and Our Obligations, New York State Journal of Medicine, April 15, 1933.
8. Arthur W. Booth, The Report of the Special Committee Appointed by the Medical Society of the State of New York to Consider the Final Report of the National Committee on the Costs of Medical Care Which Was Issued on November 29, 1933, New York State Journal of Medicine, April 15, 1933.
9. Report of the Judicial Council of the American Medical Association, Journal of the American Medical Association, May 5, 1934.
10. Douglass V. Brown, Personal communication.
11. Committee on the Costs of Medical Care, Medical Care for the American People, Final Report, Chicago, University of Chicago Press, 1932, p. 179.
12. Olin West, Discussion on Papers of Drs. White, Bass, and Cabot, Proceedings Annual Congress on Medical Education, Medical Licensure, and Hospitals, 1932.
13. Report of Special Committee, Journal of the American Medical Association, June 30, 1934.
14. Bert W. Caldwell, Opportunities of the Surgeon and the Hospital in Promoting Community Interest in the Proper Care of the Sick, Bulletin of the American College of Surgeons, December, 1933.
15. Sir Arthur Newsholme, Medicine and the State, Baltimore, Williams and Wilkins Company, 1932, p. 48.
16. Harry O. Chesley, President's Address to the New Hampshire Medical Society, New England Journal of Medicine, August 17, 1933.
17. Howard W. Haggard, The Function of the General Practitioner in Public Health Work, New England Journal of Medicine, March 15, 1934.
18. Sir Arthur Newsholme, Medicine and the State, *op. cit.*, pp. 278-79.

BIBLIOGRAPHY

BIERRING, WALTER L., The Family Doctor and the Changing Order. Journal of the American Medical Association, June 16, 1934.

This is the address of the incoming president of the American Medical Association. Dr. Bierring as a teacher, investigator, and practitioner has established for himself a deservedly high reputation.

BOOTH, ARTHUR W., The Report of the Special Committee Appointed by the Medical Society of the State of New York to Consider the Final Report of the National Committee on the Costs of Medical Care Which Was Issued on November 29, 1933. New York State Medical Journal, April 15, 1933.

This report is a satisfactory example of the current opinion of "organized medicine."

BROWN, REXWALD, The Place of Group Practice in the Development of Medicine and Hospitalization of the Future, Western Hospital Review, July, 1934.

An interesting presentation by a qualified witness.

BURGESS, MAY AYRES, Nurses, Patients, and Pocketbooks. Report of a Study of the Economics of Nursing, Conducted by the Committee on the Grading of Nursing Schools, New York, 1928.
A reliable collection of the important evidence up to that date.

CALDWELL, BERT W., Opportunities of the Surgeon and the Hospital in Promoting Community Interest in the Proper Care of the Sick. Bulletin of the American College of Surgeons, December, 1933.

This represents the official opinion of the American College of Surgeons.

CARPENTER, NILES, Medical Care for 15,000 Workers and Their Families, a Survey of the Endicott Johnson Workers Medical Service, 1928. Publication No. 5 of the Committee on the Costs of Medical Care, Chicago, University of Chicago Press, 1930.

A detailed and reliable study of medical service of the Endicott Johnson Corporation.

CLARK, EVANS, How to Budget Health, New York, Harper Brothers, 1933.

This is a study from the viewpoint of a business man. It lacks something of an understanding of the medical problems involved.

COMMISSION ON MEDICAL EDUCATION, Final Report, New York. The Commission, 1932.

This report concerns itself not only with the immediate problems to medical education, but with the whole setting of the modern practice of medicine. It contains much important factual information, and also much sound social philosophy.

COMMISSION ON MEDICAL EDUCATION, Medical Education and Related Problems in Europe, April, 1930, New York, the Commission, 1930.

Dean Rappleye, by whom this study was made for the Commission, is an experienced, well-balanced, and wise medical observer. The study is brief, but of great value.

COMMITTEE ON THE COSTS OF MEDICAL CARE, Medical Care for the American People, Chicago, University of Chicago Press, 1932.

The final report summarizes the work of this committee. The Majority Report is in some respects unsatisfactory because it attempts to reconcile the views of groups whose opinions are relatively far apart. This required an amount of compromise which prevented clear statement of the issues. It contains much that is valuable and suggestive. The first Minority Report is an excellent statement of the standpat position of "organized medicine."

COUNCIL ON MEDICAL EDUCATION AND HOSPITALS, American Medical Association. Journal of the American Medical Association, August 26, 1933.

This annual publication by the American Medical Association is a storehouse of accurate and important information.

DAVIS, MICHAEL M., Paying Your Sickness Bills, Chicago, University of Chicago Press, 1931.

Dr. Davis is a profound student of the social and economic problems of medicine. His intelligence and years of devotion to the subject entitle his opinions to great respect.

——— Change Comes to the Doctor. Survey-Graphic, April, 1934.

This shows the divergence between the social and medical opinions on the subject.

FALK, I. S., Organized Medical Service at Fort Benning, Georgia. Publication No. 21 of the Committee on the Costs of Medical Care, Chicago, University of Chicago Press, 1932.

A valuable account of the medical service offered by the United States Army Medical Corps at Fort Benning.

FALK, I. S., MARGARET C. KLEM, and NATHAN SINAI, The Incidence of Illness and the Receipt and Costs of Medical Care Among Representative Families, Experiences in Twelve Consecutive Months During 1928-1931. Publication No. 26 of the Committee on the Costs of Medical Care, Chicago, University of Chicago Press, 1933.

Gives evidence of basic value, the result of careful study.

FALK, I. S., DON M. GRISWOLD, and HAZEL I. SPICER, A Community Medical Service Organized Under Industrial Auspices in Roanoke Rapids, North Carolina. Publication No. 20 of the Committee on the Costs of Medical Care, Chicago, University of Chicago Press, 1932.
   A useful contribution to the study of Community Medical Service.

FLEXNER, ABRAHAM, Medical Education in the United States and Canada. Report of the Carnegie Foundation for the Advancement of Teaching, New York, 1910.
   The first careful study of medical education in this country. The profound changes in this field in the subsequent twenty years were largely stimulated by this book.

FOSTER, W. T., Dollars, Doctors, and Disease. Atlantic Monthly, January, 1933.
   This embodies the view of an educator and an economist. It shows some of the difficulties of reconciling the viewpoint of the economist with that of the practicing physician.

GOLDMAN and GROTJAHN, Compulsory Sickness Insurance, and, Benefits of the German Sickness Insurance System. International Labour Office of the League of Nations, 1928.
   A valuable exposition of the favorable aspects of the German system.

GRISWOLD, DON M., and HAZEL I. SPICER, University Student Health Services, a Study of Organization, Services Rendered, and Costs in Cornell University, Yale University, the University of Michigan, the University of Minnesota, the University of California, and Oregon State Agricultural College. Publication No. 19 of the Committee on the Costs of Medical Care, Chicago, University of Chicago Press, 1932.
   A trustworthy and valuable examination of some examples of university health service in 1932.

HAGGARD, HOWARD W., The Function of the General Practitioner in Public Health Work. New England Journal of Medicine, March 15, 1934.
   Dr. Haggard is Associate Professor of Applied Physiology at Yale. He brings the detachment of a scientist and appreciation of a physician to bear on the problem.

HAMILTON, WALTON H., Statement, Medical Care for the American People, Final Report of the Committee on the Costs of Medical Care, Chicago, University of Chicago Press, 1932.
   A remarkably clear statement from a profound student of social problems.

HEALTH SERVICE IN AMERICAN COLLEGES AND UNIVERSITIES, Division of Hygiene and Public Health. University of Michigan Bulletin, September 11, 1926.
   A painstaking and reliable study of University Health Service up to 1926.

HEYD, C. G., The Medical Society of the State of New York: Our Responsibilities and Our Obligations. New York State Journal of Medicine, April 15, 1933.
> This article fairly represents current medical opinion.

Hospital Number. Journal of the American Medical Association, June 11, 1932.
> This annual "Hospital" number is the best collection of data on the subject.

JOHNSON, WINGATE M., Medicine and the Middle Class. Atlantic Monthly, March, 1931.
> This states the view of an experienced practitioner of the old school.

KINGSBURY, JOHN A., Mutualizing Medical Costs. Survey-Graphic, June, 1934.
> Mr. Kingsbury speaks for the Milbank Memorial Fund. He has made a thorough study of the questions involved. His opinion is entitled to great respect.

LEE, ROGER I., and L. W. JONES, The Fundamentals of Good Medical Care, an Outline of the Fundamentals of Good Medical Care and an Estimate of the Service Required to Supply the Medical Needs of the United States. Publication No. 22 of the Committee on the Costs of Medical Care, Chicago, University of Chicago Press, 1932.
> This is the only careful attempt to estimate the amount and character of medical service which should be regarded as adequate for the present stage of medical progress. It is a very important contribution.

LELAND, R. G., Contract Practice. Journal of the American Medical Association, March 5, 1932.
> A valuable, though somewhat biased, study of contract practice.

LEVEN, MAURICE, The Income of Physicians, an Economic and Statistical Analysis. Publication No. 24 of the Committee on the Costs of Medical Care, Chicago, University of Chicago Press, 1932.
> A reliable study of this complicated subject.

LIEK, E., Die Schaden der sozialen Versicherung und Wege zur Besserung, München, J. F. Schmann Verlag, 1928.
> The defects of the German system are set forth by a competent witness.

LOWE, D. B., Industrial Health Digest, 1:2, December, 1931.
> Opinions of an expert in Industrial Medicine.

MAYERS, L., and HARRISON, L. V., The Distribution of Physicians in the United States, New York, General Medical Board, 1924.
> A very complete and careful study of this important problem. It is of basic value.

Medical Licensure Statistics for 1931. Journal of the American Medical Association, April 23, 1932.

> A most valuable collection of current facts on this subject.

Medical Relations under Workmen's Compensation. Bureau of Medical Economics, American Medical Association, Chicago, 1933.

> A valuable study from the viewpoint of organized medicine. It is based on wide study of original documents, but lacks the detachment of an unbiased observer.

MICHIGAN STATE MEDICAL SOCIETY, Official Proceedings. Supplement to Journal of the Michigan State Medical Society, May, 1934.

> A full description of an important experiment in voluntary health insurance to be set up under the auspices of a state medical society. It is based on first-hand knowledge of the British experience.

MOSER, ORAN A., The Family Doctor. New England Journal of Medicine, May 24, 1934.

> Dr. Moser is well qualified to discuss this topic.

NEWSHOLME, SIR ARTHUR, International Studies, Prevention and Treatment of Disease, Vols. I, II, III, Baltimore, Williams and Wilkins Company, 1931.

> These International Studies are a storehouse of information on social medicine in European countries and Great Britain. Sir Arthur Newsholme here sets down the results of his own recent studies. There is nowhere else to be found as complete and compact a study by so sound an observer.

——— Medicine and the State, Baltimore, Williams and Wilkins Company, 1932.

> This is the concluding volume in a series of studies made for the Milbank Memorial Fund by Sir Arthur Newsholme. He is the most experienced, and among the best qualified of English-speaking students of Medical-Social Problems. His large experience has crystallized into wisdom, and his opinions are entitled to great respect. This volume summarizes his experience, and should be read by all students of these problems.

NEWQUIST, M. N., Medical and Surgical Service in Industry and Workmen's Compensation Laws. Bulletin of the American College of Surgeons, March, 1934.

> An important contribution looking to improvement of medical service under the compensation acts.

OCHSNER, E. H., Social Insurance. Minnesota Medicine, June, 1932.

> A good example of contemporary medical opinion based on incomplete study and prejudice.

REED, LOUIS S., The Ability to Pay for Medical Care. Publication No. 25 of the Committee on the Costs of Medical Care, Chicago, University of Chicago Press, 1933.

Important and trustworthy evidence on a fundamental question.

——— The Medical Service of the Homestake Mining Company, a Survey of a Community Medical Service Operated Under Industrial Auspices. Publication No. 18 of the Committee on the Costs of Medical Care, Chicago, University of Chicago Press, 1932.

A satisfactory and unprejudiced study of medical service of the Homestake Mining Company.

Report of the Medical Service Board, American College of Surgeons, Surgery, Gynecology, and Obstetrics, July, 1934.

This report comes from qualified observers and is important.

Revue Internationale de Médicine Professionelle et Sociale, November, 1928.

Useful as showing European views of Social Medicine from a professional standpoint.

ROBB, J. M., What Shall Be the Attitude of the Physician Toward Insurance Plans? Bulletin of the American Medical Association, January, 1933.

A good example of contemporary medical opinion.

ROREM, C. RUFUS, Private Group Clinics, the Administrative and Economic Aspects of Group Medical Practice, as Represented in the Policies and Procedures of 55 Private Associations of Medical Practitioners. Publication No. 8 of the Committee on the Costs of Medical Care, Chicago, University of Chicago Press, 1931.

This is the earliest study of group practice. It is an unprejudiced report by a capable investigator. On many points it is of necessity inconclusive.

SCAMMON, RICHARD E., What Is Guild Medicine? Minnesota Medicine, March, 1933.

Dean Scammon brings to this discussion the sympathetic and detached viewpoint of a scientific observer. His opinion should command respect.

SIMONS, A. M., and NATHAN SINAI, The Way of Health Insurance, Chicago, University of Chicago Press, 1932.

This is the best study of health insurance in Europe by American observers. It is based on wide reading, and study on the ground. It lacks something of the sympathetic understanding shown by Sir Arthur Newsholme. It is, however, a most valuable book.

SINAI, NATHAN, and ALDEN B. MILLS, A Survey of the Medical Facilities of the City of Philadelphia, being in part a Digest of the Philadelphia Hospital and Health Survey, 1929. Publication No. 9 of the Committee on the Costs of Medical Care, Chicago, University of Chicago Press, 1929.

―――― A Study of Physicians and Dentists in Detroit. Publication No. 10 of the Committee on the Costs of Medical Care, Chicago, University of Chicago Press, 1929.

This, and the previous reference, are careful studies by competent observers. They provide sound statistical evidence of the facts, at the date of publication.

WALSH, WILLIAM H., The Essential Principles of the Group Purchase of Hospital Service. Bulletin of the American College of Surgeons, December, 1933.

An interesting brief statement on the important questions involved in prepayment for hospital care. Dr. Walsh speaks with the authority of knowledge.

WEISKOTTEN, H. G., Tendencies in Medical Practice. Journal of the Association of American Medical Colleges, March, 1932.

An interesting study of the tendencies toward specialization of recent medical graduates.

WEST, OLIN, The Minority Report of the Committee on the Costs of Medical Care. Minnesota Medicine, March, 1933.
This states the view of the officers of the American Medical Association.

WILLIAMS, PIERCE, The Purchase of Medical Care Through Fixed Periodic Payment, No. 20, New York, National Bureau of Economic Research, 1932.

A very complete unprejudiced presentation of a mass of facts bearing on various types of contract practice.

WHITEHEAD, ALFRED, Introduction to Wallace B. Donham, Business Adrift, New York, Whittlesey House, McGraw-Hill, 1931.

This introduction is a most enlightening and scholarly presentation of the doctrine of prediction as applied to modern conditions.

WHITE HOUSE CONFERENCE ON CHILD HEALTH AND PROTECTION, Committee on Public Health Organization, Public Health Organization, New York, The Century Company, 1932.

An important study containing much statistical data on the subject of public health organization. It also makes valuable recommendations for improvement.

INDEX

Abdomen, surgery of, rare in 1890, 7
Ability to pay for illness, 132-40; in low income groups, 205-6; in medium income groups, 206
Accidents: definition of, under Workmen's Compensation Acts, 98-99; provision for, compulsory in the Netherlands, 144; provision for, in Workmen's Compensation Acts, 97; treatment of, function of industrial medicine, 82
Advertising, spread of misinformation through, a cause of use of quacks and patent medicines, 181, 182-83
Agriculture, effects of, upon compulsory health insurance systems, 218
Alabama, industrial medical services in, 112
Alaska, medical education requirements in, 44
Alberta, limitation of supply of physicians in, 262
America, *see* United States
American College of Physicians, 52; opposed to fee-splitting, 127
American College of Surgeons, 52; opposition to fee-splitting, 126, 127; qualifications of industrial physicians listed by, 247-48; report on provision of more adequate medical service, 231-34
American Hospital Association, 230, 247, 273
American Medical Association, 244, 262; action of, on medical education, 43; actions in opposition to health insurance, 228-35; attitude toward report of American College of Surgeons, 234-35; classification and registration of specialists undertaken by, 257; development of, 252-53; *Directory* of, 257; impropriety of initiative in movement for limitation of physicians being taken by, 263; medical control of plans to distribute costs of medical care advocated by, 272; opposition to fee-splitting, 127; support of doctrine of laissez faire by, 227-35. See *also*

Bureau of Legal Medicine, Bureau of Medical Economics, Council on Medical Education and Hospitals, Judicial Council
American Society of Ophthalmologists, 52
Apothecaries' Guild, 221
Appalachian coal field, medical services in, 111-12
Appendicitis: unknown in 1890, 6
Approved Societies (British): additional medical benefits granted by, 176; relation of, to British health insurance system, 215-16; rôle of, in administration of British National Insurance Act, 167-68
Arizona, workmen's compensation in, 108-9
Arkansas, no Workmen's Compensation Act in, 105, 110
Army of the United States: community medical service provided by, in Fort Benning, Georgia, 92; remuneration in Medical Corps of, 93
Association of American Medical Colleges, 44
Association of Sickness Societies (Danish), 149
Atlantic Monthly, 224
Austria, attempt to remedy maldistribution of physicians in, 41
Automobile: effect of, upon distribution of physicians, 39; necessary expense to modern physicians, 20

Bacteriology: development of, since 1890, 14; simple in 1890, 5
Barbers' Guild, 221
Barbers of London, 50
Barthélemy, Professor, 77
Bauxite industry, medical service in, 110
Benefits, disability: effects of, in German health insurance setup, 151-52; provision for, under the British National Insurance Act, 172-74
Berlin, 153
Bierring, Dr. Walter L., 264; quoted,

Bierring, Dr. Walter L.—*Continued*
on limitation of supply of physicians, 262-63
Binghamton, New York, 84, 85
Bismarck von Schönhausen, Otto von, 150
Blood, knowledge of, increased since 1890, 15
Booth, Arthur W., 267
Botanics, 51
British Empire, registration general in, 50
British Hospital Savings Association, 210
British Medical Association, 215; function of, in disciplining physicians, 255-56; opinions of, regarding the British health insurance system, 174-75; part played by, in development of compulsory health insurance, 161; proposals by, to extend the British health insurance system, 177; relationships of, to health insurance system, 166-67, 168, 169
British National Insurance Act, 166-72
Brown, Professor Douglass V., 270
Brown, Dr. Rexwald, 258; quoted, on group practice, 73-75; quoted, on opposition to group practice, 244
Bruce, Dr. J. D., 229
Bureau of Legal Medicine, 253
Bureau of Medical Economics, 230, 253; quoted, on free choice of physicians, 100, 256-57
Business, trend towards professionalization of, 31-32

California: licensure in, 51; supply of physicians in, 35
California Industrial Accident Commission, 98
Calumet and Hecla Consolidated Copper Company, medical services of, 110
Canada: attempt to reduce maldistribution of physicians in, 200-201; handling of workmen's compensation insurance funds in, 97; limitation of supply of physicians in, 262; minimum income guaranteed to rural physicians by, 280; rural physicians subsidized in, 179; supply of medical schools in, 44, 45
Cary, Dr. E. H., 229
Carnegie Foundation for the Advancement of Teaching, 43
Charles River, appearance of malaria along, in 1890, 7
Chemistry: aid to pharmacology, 15-16; aid to physiology, 16; development of, since 1890, 17-18; simple in 1890, 5
Chesley, Dr. Harry O., 274-75
Child health: American program for, 185-87; value of a program for improvement of, 278
Children, incidence of illness among, 138; specialist needed for care of, 193
China, contract practice in, 105
Chiropractors, distribution of, 40
Choice of physician, *see* Free choice of physicians
Church, learned professions originated from, 120
Cities, conditions of medical practice in, 61-62
Civil service: bad conditions in United States affecting public health officers, 184; British principle of, 159; effects upon medical service in Great Britain, 162; importance of, to good stystem of compulsory health insurance, 218-20
Clinics, supply of, 46
"Cloak of mystery": necessary in 1890, 6; no longer defensible, 22
College education, prerequisite to medical education, 18
Colorado, workmen's compensation in, 108-9
Colorado Iron and Fuel Company, elaborate medical service of, 109
Commission on Medical Education, 260; final report quoted, 44-45
Committee on the Costs of Medical Care, 72, 153, 207, 210, 237; American Medical Association's criticism of *Majority Report* of, 227-28; *Minorty Report* of, 69, 73, 77; *Minority Report* of, quoted, on medical control of plans to distribute costs of medical care, 271
Communication, changes in, 29
Community health, needs for, in United States, 183-85
Community medical services, 90-93; long-time medical planning possibilities of, 242-43
Competition: effects of, in Great Britain, prior to establishment of British Compulsory Insurance System, 165; effects of, on medical practice, 259-60; evil influence of, in respect to contract

INDEX

Competition—*Continued*
practice, 250-51; limitation of number of physicians in conflict with doctrine of, 261; medical problems arising from, 128-31; summary of views concerning, 282

Compulsion: methods of, in Denmark's health insurance setup, 148; public opinion limits use of, in United States, 239

Connecticut Board of Compensation Commissioners, quoted, on free choice of physicians, 100

Consultations, financial consideration regarding, 60-61

Contagious disease, value of public health service in diminishing, 183

Contract practice: Danish health insurance system calls for, 149; long-time medical planning possibilities of, 250-51; medical groups as entering into, 72; provided by British Friendly Societies, 167; under Workmen's Compensation Acts, 104-6

Copenhagen, 145, 148, 149

Cornell University, health service at, 79-80

Cost of medical care: ability to pay for, 132-40; amount of, under the British National Insurance Act, 172; control of plans to distribute, 271-76; distribution of ability to pay for, 134-38; doctrine of laissez faire as applied to, 225; group practice leads to reduction of, 76-77; Homestake Mine Medical service costs, 87; in Fort Benning, Georgia, 92-93; in Germany, *Krankenkassen* try to keep down, 154; in Roanoke Rapids, North Carolina, 91; low income groups' ability to pay for, 205-6; medium income groups' ability to pay for, 206; university health services, 80

Council on Medical Education and Hospitals, 252, 262

County medical societies: offering of medical service by, 212; voluntary health insurance under auspices of, 244-46

Crookshank, Dr., 225

Cults, licensure problems due to existence of, 52-54

Danish Medical Association, 147; contracts with Association of Sickness Societies, 149

Davis, Michael M., 86, 229

Delft, 143

Denmark: long-existing conditions necessary to development of health insurance in, 240; results of voluntary health insurance in, 208-9; supply of physicians in, 38; voluntary health insurance in, 145-48

Dental care: an additional benefit granted by the British Approved Societies, 176; extension of, important for program of preventive medicine, 187; offering of, by medical groups, 71; school health programs as attacking neglect of, 186-87

Dentists: adequacy of supply of, in United States, 201-2; collection of fees by, 117; supervision of, in Denmark, 145; supply of, in United States, 186-87

Detroit, 153; proportion of specialists in, 61

Diagnosis: care in, unprofitable to *Krankenkassen* physicians, 156; complexity of, factor in growth of hospitals, 34; difficult in 1890, 10; internists' function in, 64-65; methods of, in 1890, 5-6; modern requirements of, 21-34; now a complicated affair, 21; physics as an aid to, 17; scientific aids to, 14-18; value of family characteristics in, 11

Diphtheria: little understood in 1890, 6

Directory of the American Medical Association, information as to qualifications of physicians given by, 257

Disability benefits, *see* Benefits, disability

Discipline: inability of organized medicine to achieve, 255-56; public interest must be safeguarded in subjecting physicians to, 281-82

Discoveries, medical ethics require making available of, 252-53

Distribution of medical service: physicians, 38-43. *See also* Highlands and Islands Medical Service, Rural areas, Physicians

District of Columbia, medical education requirements in, 44

Doctors, *see* Physicians

Drugs, *see* Pharmacology

304 INDEX

Eclecticism, 51

Economic conditions: as limiting use of modern transportation and communication, 30; changes in, slow until 1870, 3; compulsory health insurance schemes must take account of, 217; effects of, upon disability benefits in Great Britain, 173; effects upon amount of medical service, 138-40; effects upon group practice of medicine, 73, 76-77; important changes in last forty years, 9-12

Edison Electric Illuminating Company of Boston, 138

Education, high level of, in United States, 181

Employees, unsatisfactory position of, under liability laws, 94-95. *See also* Workmen's Compensation Acts

Endicott, New York, 84, 85

Endicott Johnson Corporation, medical service provided by, 84-86

Endicott Johnson Workers Medical Service, 84-86

Engineering, salaries as basis of payment in, 131

England (and Wales): civil service in, a condition making for success of compulsory health insurance, 219; condition of medical service in, prior to establishment of British Compulsory Insurance System, 164-66; discussion of compulsory health insurance in, 213-16; Friendly Societies paved way for compulsory health insurance in, 240; group practice, new development in, 77; growth of voluntary health insurance in, 238; history of guilds in, 221; hospital insurance, a success in, 246; hospital insurance in, 210; leader in workmen's compensation legislation, 94; medical service in, 158-76; methods of disciplining physicians in, 255-56; proportion of specialists in, 196; provision of medical care for medium income groups in, 206; school hygiene less developed in the United States than in, 277; sharp division between specialists and general practitioners in, 258; supply of physicians in, 38; use of midwives customary in, 89

Ethics, codes of, 57; accepted practices of a commercial age in conflict with, 126-27

Examinations, periodic, utility of, doubted, 187-89

Experience, not as great an asset to physician as formerly, 25

Eye, diseases of, general practitioner cannot treat, 193

Family: no longer unit of medical care, 195

Family doctor: advantages of, 10-11; advantages of, severely curtailed today, 24-25; counsellor on many non-medical questions, 12; defense of, 226; impossibility of resurrection of, 191, 195; opinions of, unsupported by accurate data, 21. *See also* General practitioners

Farmers, changes in status of, 32-33

Federal Liability Law, 106

Fees: collection of, 116-17; problem of, complicated by donating of charity medical services, 267-71; problems concerning, 119-25; sliding scale of, discussed, 121-23. *See also* Fee-splitting, Remuneration, Sliding scale of fees

Fee-splitting: discussion of, 125-28; informal group practice as solution of, 197; prevalence of, 127-28; reasons for, 60-61

"Fellow servant," doctrine of, 94

Finance, questions of, regarding consultations, 60

Flexner, Dr. Abraham, 43

Florida, no Workmen's Compensation Act in, 105

Fort Benning, Georgia, 140; community medical service in, 92-93

Forum, 225

Foster, Professor Nellis B., 86, 237

Framingham, Massachusetts, ability to pay for medical care in, 136

France: supply of physicians in, 38; unsatisfactory development of organized medicine in, 77

Free choice of physicians: British health insurance system provides for, 171, 215; difficulties of, discussed, 58-59; discussion of doctrine of, 256-59; Netherlands' health insurance makes no provision for, 144; provision for, by Great Western Railway Medical Fund Society,

Free choice of physicians—*Continued*
89-90; status under workmen's compensation acts, 99-101
Friendly Societies (British): British compulsory health insurance system grew from care provided by, 240; medical care provided by, prior to establishment of British Compulsory Insurance System, 165; rôle of, under British National Insurance Act, 167-68

General Medical Council (British), 160-61, 266, 281; function of, in disciplining physicians, 255-56
General practitioners: as successors to family doctors, 25; competence of, to carry out periodic health examinations, doubted, 189; complicated diagnostic methods must be accessible to, 24; contrast of income, with specialists, 116; diagnosis and assignment of specialists greatest services of, 25; difficulty of determining qualifications of, 257-58; impossibility of keeping up-to-date, 226; income of, 63; internists as modern development of, 65; knowledge required of, 27-28; modern training of, 19; needs in respect to, in United States, 190-95; obligations of, 55-57; problems faced by, 57-63; scientific methods of diagnosis not available to, in 1890, 11-12; temptation to perform specialized work, 124. *See also* Family doctors
Genito-urinary tract: complicated examinations necessary in diseases of, 23-24; diseases of, specialist needed for adequate diagnosis and treatment, 193-94
Germany: compulsory health insurance in, 104, 149-57; discussion of compulsory health insurance in, 213-16; proportion of specialization in, 196; supply of physicians in, 38
Glasgow, 178
Goldman, Dr., 157
Government: British system of, 158-59; medical care of indigent, a responsibility of, 269; medical care of indigent by, condemned by Judicial Council of the American Medical Association, 268-69; medical supervision by, in Denmark, 145-46; supervision of medical care by, in Great Britain, 159-62

Government hospitals: in Great Britain, 163-164; supply and use of, 45-46. *See also* State hospitals
Graduates, medical, supply and training of, 43-45
Great Britain, *see* England (and Wales), Scotland
Great Western Railway Medical Fund Society, services provided by, 88-90
Grotjahn, Dr., 157
Group health services, 79-93
Group practice, 68-78; evil competitive practices minimized by, 129; informal, solution of problem of fee-splitting, 197; long-time medical planning possibilities of, 243-44; offering of health insurance in connection with, 211-12; university health service as example of, 79-81. *See also* Group health services
Guild medicine: not a desirable development, 220-23
Guilds, history of, 220-21
Gynecologists, certification of, 52

Haggard, Dr. Howard W., 275-76
Halifax Paper Company, 90
Hamilton, Walton H., quoted, on compulsory health insurance, 237; quoted, on free choice of physicians, 58-59
Harvard, 55
Health, accurate diagnosis essential to care of, 21
Health education, a function of university health services, 81
Health insurance: American Medical Association's opposition to, 228-35; as a means of improving medical service in the United States, 207-20; British National Insurance Act, 166-72; compulsory, applicability of, to United States, 216-20; compulsory, as method of improving medical service in the United States, 237-40; compulsory, in Germany, 149-57; compulsory, in the British Isles, 158-79; concern for indigent, a cause of weakness in, 166; in Europe, 141-79; possible coexistence of compulsory and voluntary systems of, 177; provision for medical care by hospitals, 246; regular life and accident insurance companies do not offer, 209-10; value of, for medium income groups, 206; voluntary, in the Netherlands,

Health insurance—*Continued*
142-45; voluntary, remarkable unanimity as to futility of, 238; voluntary, under auspices of county medical societies, 244-46
Hematology, development of, since 1890, 15
Heyd, C. G., 267
Highlands and Islands Medical Service, 178-79; a solution of problem of maldistribution of physicians, 200, 280
Holland, *see* Netherlands
Homeopathy, 51
Homestake Mine Medical Service, 86-88
Homestake Mining Company, medical service offered by, 86-88
Hooker, Professor Ransom S., 86
Hospitals: charity support of, decreasing, 272-73; contract system in West Virginia coal fields, 112-13; development of group practice around, 70; development of informal group practice around, 197; diseases of, in 1890, 8; examples of group practice, 68; growth in number, size, and use of, 33-34; health insurance by, 246-47; inadequacies in supply of, in United States, 202-3; need for, in modern medical practice, 20; offering of insurance plans by, 210-11; out-patient departments of, 46; payment to, under Workmen's Compensation Acts, 102-3; social service, a modern development of, 34; state of development in 1890, 7-9; status of, in Germany, 152-53; supervision of, in Denmark, 145; supply of, in Denmark, 146; supply of, in Great Britain, 162-64; supply of, in the Netherlands, 144; supply of, in the United States, 45-47. *See also* Government hospitals, Private hospitals, State hospitals

Idaho, workmen's compensation in, 108-9
Illinois, workmen's compensation in, 109-10
Illness: duration of, increases under health insurance, 155-56; incidence of, 138-40
Immunization, child health program as aid to, 186
Income: national distribution of, 134; of physicians, *see* Remuneration
Income tax: charity contributions to hospitals reduced by increase in, 273; sliding scale of fees as, 123
Indiana, workmen's compensation in, 109-10
Indigent: British voluntary hospitals originally intended for care of, 163; care of, effect upon basis for fees, 123-24; care of, in the Netherlands, 142-43; charity medical service as a method of caring for, 266-71; concern for, cause of weaknesses in health insurance systems, 166; county medical societies' attempts to care for, 212; hospital social service intended for, 34; inadequacies in medical care for, in United States, 203-4; official medical assistance for, in Great Britain, 164; summary of views concerning care of, 282
Individualism: of physicians, must be considered in group plans, 212; relation of group practice to, 76
Industrial medicine: contract medicine developed in connection with, 105; development of, 81-90; future possibilities of, 247-49; reasons for development of, 30-31
Industrial Revolution, cause of need for Workmen's Compensation Acts, 94
Industry: changes in, 30-32; changes in, a cause of Workmen's Compensation Acts, 94; hazards and diseases of, a recent development, 9; medical efforts of, criticized by medical profession, 83; qualifications for industrial physicians required by, 248
Infection: control of, a factor in growth of hospitals, 33; Listerian doctrine not fully developed in 1890, 7; surgeons as a cause of, in 1890, 8-9
Injury, *see* Accidents
Insurance, *see* Health insurance
Insurance carriers: actions under liability laws, 95; difficulties of Workmen's Compensation Acts due to creation of, 241-42; functions under Workmen's Compensation Acts, 96-97; payment for medical services by, 101-2; rôle of, in administration of British National Insurance Act, 167-68; selection of physicians by, 99-101
International Labor Office, 153
International Medical Association, quoted, on free choice of physicians, 100

Internists, functions of, 64-65
Iowa, workmen's compensation in, 109-10

Jefferson Medical College of Philadelphia, 55
Johns Hopkins, 55
Johnson, Dr. Wingate M., 226
Johnson City, New York, 84, 85
Journal of the American Medical Association, 227
Judicial Council, 234, 252; definition of contract practice by, 104-5; function of, in disciplining of members by the American Medical Association, 255; report on government medical care for the indigent, 268-69
Julius Rosenwald Fund, 86
Jutland, 148

Kansas, workmen's compensation in, 109-10
Kentucky, industrial medical services in, 112; licensure in, 51
Kingsbury, John A., 237
Krankenkassen: complete medical care offered by, 151; conflict with medical profession, 153; development of, 150-51; hospitals operated by, 152; relation of, to physicians, 154-57; relationship to physicians and patients, 216; similarity of British Approved Societies to, 176

Labor, compulsory health insurance opposed by, 216, 240
Laboratories, need of modern medical practice, 20
Laissez faire, doctrine of: American Medical Association's support of, 227-35; application of, to medical practice, 224-37
Lake Superior iron mining industry, medical service in, 110
Law, status of compensation in, previous to Workmen's Compensation Acts, 95
Lawyers, *see* Legal profession
Laymen: ability of, to select physicians, 58-59; representation of, in medical groups, a means of maintaining contact with public opinion, 274-76
Lead, South Dakota, 86
League of Red Cross Societies, 154
Legal profession: classification of lawyers by, 258-59; problem of fees not difficult in, 120; salaries as basis of payment in, 130-31
Legislation: obligation of physicians in regard to, 53; relation of medical profession to, Workmen's Compensation Acts, 98-99
Leland, Dr. R. G., 229
Leven, Maurice, 117
Lewis, F., 173
Licensure, history and problems of, 50-54
Liek, Dr. E., 157
Limitation of number of physicians: discussed, 260-66; summary of views on, 282. *See also* Supply of physicians
Lister, Joseph, 7, 33
Lloyd George, David, 166, 168
London, supply of hospitals in, 162-63
Long Island College of Medicine, 55
Los Angeles County Medical Society, statement of, on number of persons lacking medical aid, 236
Lowe, Dr. Don B., 83
Low income groups: compulsory health insurance in Germany improved medical service to, 214; inadequacy of medical care of, in the United States, 205-6
Lumbering, contract practice highly developed in, 105

Maladjustments: family doctor as assistant in those not due to disease conditions, 12
Malaria, cause of, unknown in 1890, 7
Martindale-Hubbel Law Directory, 258
Maryland, 112
Massachusetts, first to have workmen's compensation laws, 94
Massachusetts Medical Society, licensure by, 50-51
Master Barbers Association, 50
Maternity, German benefits for medical care in, 152
Mayo Clinic, 70
Medical Corps of the Army of the United States, remuneration in, 93
Medical education: description of, in 1890, 4; discussion of criticisms of, 26-27; factor in maldistribution of physicians, 40, 41; modern requirements for, 18-20; needs for, in regard to specialists, 197-98; possibility of limiting supply of physicians through control of,

Medical education—*Continued*
261-65; provision for, in Denmark, 147; quality and supply of, 43-45; requirements for specialists, 66, 67; requirements of, 44; vast improvement in, in thirty years, 279

Medical Education in the United States and Canada, 43

Medical practice, changing conditions of, factor in the distribution of physicians, 39-40; contrast between that in 1890 and that in 1930, 3-20; general, 50-63; specialization not peculiar to, 64. *See also* Contract practice, Group practice

Medical profession, *see* Organized medicine

Medical schools: function of, in university health services, 79-80; supply of, in the United States, 43-44

Medical service: ability to pay for, 132-40; distribution of ability to pay for, 134-38; great potential improvement of, in the United States, 279-83; improvement of, must be based on local conditions, 180

Medical Society of the State of New York: report on charity medical services, 267-68

Medium income groups, inadequacy of medical care for, in the United States, 206

Men, incidence of illness among, 138

Mental hygiene, Yale health service provision for, 80

Miasms, regarded as causes of yellow fever and malaria, 6-7

Michigan, workmen's compensation in, 109-10

Michigan copper mining field, medical service in, 110

Michigan State Medical Society, 245; investigation of health insurance plans by, 228-30

Middle West, development of group practice in, 70

Midwives: (Denmark) education of, 147, 149; supervision of, 145; (Great Britain) education and supervision of, 177-78; (Netherlands) function of, 145. *See also* Obstetrical care

Milwaukee, 230

Mining: coal, medical service in, 109; contract practice highly developed in, 105. *See also* Appalachian coal field, Lake Superior iron mining industry, Michigan copper mining field

Ministry of Health (British), 159-60, 215; description of, 169-70; public health supervision by, 161-62; rôle of, in administration of British National Insurance Act, 169, 174

Mississippi, no workmen's compensation act in, 105

Missouri, workmen's compensation in, 109-10

Mobility of population, effects of, on medical practice, 29

Monopoly: guilds as a method of, 221; supervised and controlled, indicated for the future, 129; tendency for medical practice to acquire aspects of, 265

Montana, workmen's compensation in, 108-9

Moser, Dr. Oran A., 226

Muller, George P., 93

Nashville, 230

National Board of Medical Examiners, 51-52

National Conference of Friendly Societies, 173

National Insurance Gazette, 173

Negligence, contributory, doctrine of, 94

Netherlands, health insurance in, 142-45

Nevada, workmen's compensation in, 108-9

New England, bills for medical service formerly rarely rendered in, 120

New Hampshire, licensure in, 51

New Hampshire Medical Society, 51, 274

New Jersey, licensure in, 50

Newman, Sir George, 166, 170, 219

New Mexico, workmen's compensation in, 108-9

Newsholme, Sir Arthur, 142; quoted, on effects of British National Insurance Act, 175-76; quoted, on free choice of physicians, 257; quoted, on group medical practice, 73; quoted, on hospitals in Denmark, 146; quoted, on medical secrecy, 77; quoted, on public control of plans to distribute the costs of medical care, 273-74; quoted, on school hygiene in the United States, 278

New York (State): licensure in, 51;

INDEX 309

New York (State)—*Continued*
workmen's compensation legislation in, 97
Noblesse oblige, doctrine of, responsible for development of British voluntary hospital system, 162
North Carolina, supply of physicians in, 35
Northwest, development of group practice in, 70
Norway, supply of physicians in, 38
Nurses, trained: adequacy of supply of, in United States, 201; income of, 48; supply meager in 1890, 10; supply of, 47-49. *See also* Nursing
Nursing: institutional, 49; private duty, 48-49. *See also* Nurses, trained; Public health nursing

Obstetrical care: British health insurance system does not provide for, 171; British provision for, 177-78; Great Western Railway Medical Fund provides for, 89; provision for, in the Netherlands, 145. *See also* Midwives
Obstetricians, certification of, 52
Occupational disease, medical aspects of, 83
Ohio: example of satisfactory relation between medical profession and industrial commission, 104; industrial medical services in, 112
Oklahoma, workmen's compensation in, 109-10
Old age insurance: in Germany, 150; instrument of compulsion in Denmark, 148; part of British National Insurance Act, 167; universal in Denmark, 149
Operations, *see* Surgery
Ophthalmic treatment, an additional benefit granted by the British Approved Societies, 176
Ophthalmologists, certification of, 52
Oregon, workmen's compensation in, 108
Oregon Agricultural College, health service at, 79-80
Organized medicine: conflict with *Krankenkassen*, in Germany, 153; contract medical service opposed by, 72; control by, of plans for distributing the cost of medical care, 271-76; criticism of industrialists by, 83; development of, 252-55; disregard of public opinion by, dangerous, 78; fee-splitting opposed by, 126-27; group practice opposed by, 244; hospital insurance opposed by, 246-47; indifferent to enactment of Workmen's Compensation Acts, 96; likely to promote development of medical syndicalism, 77; need for assumption of responsibility for selection of workmen's compensation physicians by, 101; not a guild, 221-23; plans for voluntary health insurance not encouraged by, 242; position of, concerning legislation, 53-54; power of, to control and discipline its members, insufficient to correct evils, 251; relation to compensation acts, 103-4; school health programs opposed by, 185-86; suggestions for future guidance of, summarized, 280-81. *See also* American College of Surgeons, American Medical Association, British Medical Association, Committee on the Costs of Medical Care, County medical societies, Danish Medical Association, International Medical Association, Los Angeles County Medical Society, Medical Society of the State of New York, Michigan State Medical Society, Wayne County Medical Society
Orthopedists, necessary training of, 66
Out-patient departments of hospitals, increasing use of, 46
Overhead: group practice reduction of, 69; large proportion of physicians' gross income, 20
Owego, New York, 84

Pacific States, supply of physicians in, 35
Pasteur, Louis, 33
Patent medicines, advertising an aid to, 181
Pathology, development of, since 1890, 14-15
Patients: free choice of physicians not demanded by, 256; psychology of, a problem in utilization of periodic health examinations, 188-89; relation of, with physicians, must be personal, 190; status of, improved under German health insurance, 156. *See also* Free choice of physicians, Laymen, Personal

310 INDEX

Patients—*Continued*
  relation between patient and physician, Public
Patterson Mills Company, 90
Pennsylvania: ability to pay for medical care in, 136; industrial medical services in, 112
Personal relationship between patient and physician, influence of group practice upon, 71-72
Pharmacology, development of, since 1890, 15-16
Philadelphia, proportion of specialists in, 61
Physical examination: changes in methods of, 22-23; industrial medicine provision for, 82; university health services provide for, 81
Physicians: charity medical service in relation to income of, 266-71; collection of fees by, 116-17; competition among, in Great Brtain, prior to establishment of the British Compulsory Insurance System, 165; defining of injury and accident by, under Workmen's Compensation Acts, 98-99; distribution of income in private practice, 114-18; doctrine of laissez faire held by many, 224; effects of development of science upon, 12-18; inability to give time to committees a handicap to organized medicine, 254; individualism of, notorious, 212; knowledge required of, in 1890, 4; modern equipment of, 18-20; poor collection of fees by, 116-17; public interference with, undesirable, 23; radius of action, factors increasing, 30; radius of action small in 1890, 10; relation of, to *Krankenkassen*, 154-57; short working life of, 117-18; status of in Germany, 153-57; subsidizing of, in rural areas, by Scotland, 179; supervision of, in Denmark, 145; use of hospital facilities by, 47. *See also* Family doctors, General practitioners, Specialists, Supply of physicians
Physics, aid to medicine, 17
Physiology: aid to pharmacology, 15; development of, since 1890, 16
Politics, effects of, upon public health service, 184
Poor, the, *see* Indigent
Poor Law Hospitals (British), 164

Population: mobility of, a factor in compulsory health insurance, 218; shifts in distribution of, during last forty years, 9; shifts of, statistics cited, 28-29
Prepayment plans, *see* Health insurance
Preventive medicine: essential requirement of today, 18; needs for, in United States, 185-90; present amount of medical service inadequate for, 140
Private hospitals, supply and use of, 45-46
Private practice, distribution of income among physicians in, 114-18
Profession, medical, *see* Organized medicine
Professions, public obligations of, 56-57. *See also* Dentists, Engineering, Legal profession, Organized medicine
Profit: care of the health of the community not proper subject for, 241-42; contract medicine made difficult by considerations of, 250
Prussia, 150
Public: failure of, to take expert advice, a cause of blunders, 22; lack of adequate medical equipment, responsibility of, 21; limitation in number of physicians would affect interests of, 265-66; rights of, as consumers of medical service, 78; rights of, in control of plans to distribute the cost of medical care, 272-76
Public health nursing: extension of, desirable, 277; supply of, 49
Public health services: conditions affecting, in United States, 183-85; necessity for extension of, 277-78; permanent medical committees required by organized medicine for effective influence on, 253-54
Public opinion: an unsound and risky control of medical practice, 22; questions regarding group practice must be decided by, 78; relation of group practice to, 77; use of compulsion limited by, 239

Quacks, advertising an aid to, 181

Railroads, workmen's compensation relating to, 105-6
Redistribution of wealth, charity con-

Redistribution of wealth—*Continued*
tributions to hospitals will be reduced by, 273
Registration: control of physicians' qualification by, in Great Britain, 160-61; history of, in England, 50
Remuneration: charity medical service in relation to, 266-71; from insurance carriers, 101-2; increased and stabilized by British health insurance system, 215; in Denmark, 148-49; in Endicott Johnson Workers Medical Service, 85-86; in England (and Wales), under British health insurance system, 172; in Germany, 153-54; in Great Western Railway Medical Fund Society, 89; in Homestake Mine Medical Service, 87; in Medical Corps of the Army of the United States, 93; in Roanoke Rapids, North Carolina, 91; in the United States, 114-31; of general practitioners, 63; of nurses, 48; of specialists, 67-68; salary basis for, desirable, 282. *See also* Fees, Salaries
Research, a function of specialists, 26
Resources, medical, 35-49
Riesman, Professor David, 93
Risk, doctrine of assumption of, 94
Rist, Dr., 77
Roanoke Mills Company, 90
Roanoke Rapids, North Carolina, 243; community medical service in, 90-92
Rochester, New York, ability to pay for medical care in, 136
Roosevelt, Franklin D., 246
Rosemary Manufacturing Company, 90
Ross-Loos Clinic: attempt to reduce maldistribution of physicians, 201; health insurance offered by, 211
Royal College of Physicians, 50
Royal College of Surgeons, 50; practice of surgery limited to members of, 258
Royal Commission on National Health Insurance, 174
Royal Commission on the Poor Laws, report of, responsible for the British health insurance system, 166
Rural areas; necessary equipment of modern physicians in, 20; plans for insuring adequate medical service in, 279-83; problems of medical service in, 40, 42-43; subsidizing of physicians in, as a method of improving medical service, 179

Salaries: basis of payment, in hospitals of Denmark, 146; desirability of incomes based upon, 282; income of physicians working for, 118-19; payment on basis of, discussed, 130-31. *See also* Remuneration
Sand, Dr. René, 154
Saskatchewan, Province of, attempt to reduce maldistribution of physicians in, 200-1
Savings, as a means for paying for medical care, 137-38
Scammon, Professor Richard E., 221
School health services: as aid to a program of preventive medicine, 185-87; need for extension of, 277-78
Science: American people interested in, 181-82; amount of, underlying medical practice, not great in 1890, 4; increase in knowledge of, a cause of specialization, 64; tremendous development of, since 1890, 12-18
Scotland: provision of medical service in, 178-79; subsidy to rural physicians by, 280
Scrofula, prevalent in 1890, 7
Simons, A. M., 153, 236
Sinai, Nathan, 61, 153, 236
Sliding scale of fees: propriety of, questioned by Texas court decision, 270; reasons for development of, 121-23; relation of charity medical services to, 267; theory of, open to question, 269-70
Small towns, conditions of medical practice in, 62
Social conditions: changes in, slow before 1870, 3; important changes in, in last forty years, 9-12
Social insurance: in Germany, 150
Socialized medicine, *see* Group practice, Health insurance
Social service, hospital, a modern development, 34
South Atlantic states, supply of physicians in, 35
South Carolina: no workmen's compensation act in, 105; supply of physicians in, 35
Specialists: assignment of, duty of gen-

Specialists—*Continued*
eral practitioner, 25; certification of, 52; contrast of income of, with income of general practitioners, 116; expensive equipment essential to, 20; few in 1890, 4; income of, 67-68; long preparation necessary for, 19; necessary training for, 66; needs relating to, in United States, 195-98; research a function of, 26; services of, must be freely available to general practitioners, 24. *See also* Specialization

Specialization, 64-68; development of, gone further in this country, 182; effects upon distribution of physicians, 39; extent and reasons for, 25-28; growth of, 54-55; growth of, cause of fee-splitting, 126; increase in medical costs due to, 225; problem of fees complicated by, 122-23; result of forces making for subdivision of labor, 64; scientific developments, a force making for increase in, 18. *See also* Industrial medicine, Specialists

State hospitals, bed occupancy in, 46

States, inadequacy of, as units for compulsory health insurance systems, 217-18

Stethoscope, use of, in 1890, 5

Students, difficulty in proper selection of, 264-65

Supply of physicians: adequacy of, in the United States, 35-38, 198-99; distribution of, 38-43; limitation of, discussed, 260-66; maldistribution of, problems related to, 199-201. *See also* Limitation of supply of physicians

Supreme Court of Wisconsin, 98

Surgeons: cause of infection in 1890, 8-9; practice of, in 1890, 4-5

Surgery: financial temptation to perform unnecessary operations, 125; increase in amount of, a factor in growth of hospitals, 33-34; poorly developed in 1890, 7; practice of, restricted in Great Britain, 258; problem of fees complicated by development of, 122-23; specialists needed for, 193; specialization in, greatest, 65-66; undertaken in private homes in 1890, 8

Sweden: limitation of physicians in, 260; supply of physicians in, 38

Swindon, Wiltshire County, England, group medical service in, 88-90

Syphilis, management of, a specialty, 65. *See also* Venereal diseases

Telephone: aid to rural medical service, 42; necessary expense to modern physician, 20

Tennessee, industrial medical services in, 112

Tenure of office of public health officials, effects of, upon medical service in Great Britain, 162. *See also* Civil service, Public health services

Texas: licensure in, 51; sliding scale questioned by court decision in, 270

Therapeutics, physics as an aid to, 17

Thomsonianism, 51

Transportation: changes in, 29; changes in, since 1890, 9-10; effects of, upon compulsory health insurance systems, 218; effects of, upon distribution of physicians, 39, 42

Treatment, medical, complexity of, factor in growth of hospitals, 34

Tuberculosis: contributions to care of, in Germany, 152; not readily diagnosed in 1890, 6; specialist needed for diagnosis of, 193

Tufts College Medical School, 55

Typhoid fever, frequency of, great in 1890, 6

United States: applicability of compulsory health insurance to, 216-20; capacity of, to deliver a superior medical service, 279-83; cost of illness in, 133; development of group practice peculiar to, 76; history of licensure in, 50-52; history of Workmen's Compensation Acts in, 94-96; industrial accidents in, 97; lack of high-grade civil service in, a handicap to possibility of compulsory health insurance, 220; measures of compulsion inapplicable to, 239; medical needs in, 180-206; medical resources of, 35-49; possibility of subsidizing rural physicians in, 179; prerequisite conditions for development of compulsory health insurance do not exist in, 209; probable value of voluntary health insurance in, 212; proportion of specialists in, 196; school hy-

INDEX 313

United States—*Continued*
giene more developed in Great Britain than in, 277; special conditions in, require special measures, 180-82; supply of hospital beds in, 46; supply of medical schools in, 44. *See also* Army of the United States

United States Public Health Service, 184

Universities, hospitals of, in Germany, 152-53

University and Bellevue Hospital Medical College, 55

University health service, 79-81

University of California, health service at, 79-80

University of Cologne, 152

University of Hamburg, 152

University of Michigan, health service at, 79-80

University of Minnesota, health service at, 79-80

University of Pennsylvania, 50

Urologists, necessary training of, 66

Utah, workmen's compensation in, 108-9

Venereal disease: money benefits for medical care of, in Germany, 152; specialist needed for treatment of, 194. *See also* Syphilis

Vermont, licensure in, 51

Virginia, industrial medical services in, 112

Virginia Electric and Power Company, 90

Waiting period, effects of, in workmen's compensation, 97

Walsh, Dr. William H., 246

Washington, D. C., *see* District of Columbia

Washington (State), workmen's compensation in, 107-8

Wayne County Medical Society, quoted, in opposition to health insurance, 245

Way of Health Insurance, The, 153

West, Dr. Olin, 228, 229

West North Central states, supply of physicians in, 35

West Virginia: ability to pay for medical care in, 136; hospital contract system in, 112-13; industrial medical services in, 112

Whitehead, Alfred, 3

Women, incidence of illness among, 138

Woodward, Dr. William C., 229

Workmen's Compensation Acts: contract practice stimulated by, 105; effects of, upon medical practice, 94-113; industrial medicine based upon requirements of, 247; influence in formation of Endicott Johnson Workers Medical Service, 84; lessons of, to long-time medical planning, 240-42; stimulus to development of industrial medicine, 81-82

World War: alteration in medical outlook due to, 190; effects of, upon British hospitals, 163; effects of, upon health insurance in Germany, 154-55; impetus to development of group practice, 70

Wyoming, medical service in, 109

X rays: excessive use of, demanded by patients, 22; necessary in physicial examinations, 23; need for, in modern medical practice, 20; use in diagnosis and therapeutics, 17; use in physiology, 16

Yale University, health service at, 79-80

Yellow fever, frequency of, great in 1890, 6

COLUMBIA UNIVERSITY PRESS
COLUMBIA UNIVERSITY
NEW YORK

FOREIGN AGENT
OXFORD UNIVERSITY PRESS
HUMPHREY MILFORD
AMEN HOUSE, LONDON, E.C. 4

Bei Fragen zur Produktsicherheit wenden Sie sich bitte an:
If you have any questions regarding product safety,
please contact:

Walter de Gruyter GmbH
Genthiner Straße 13
10785 Berlin
productsafety@degruyterbrill.com